HANDBOOK OF MEDICAL ACUPUNCTURE

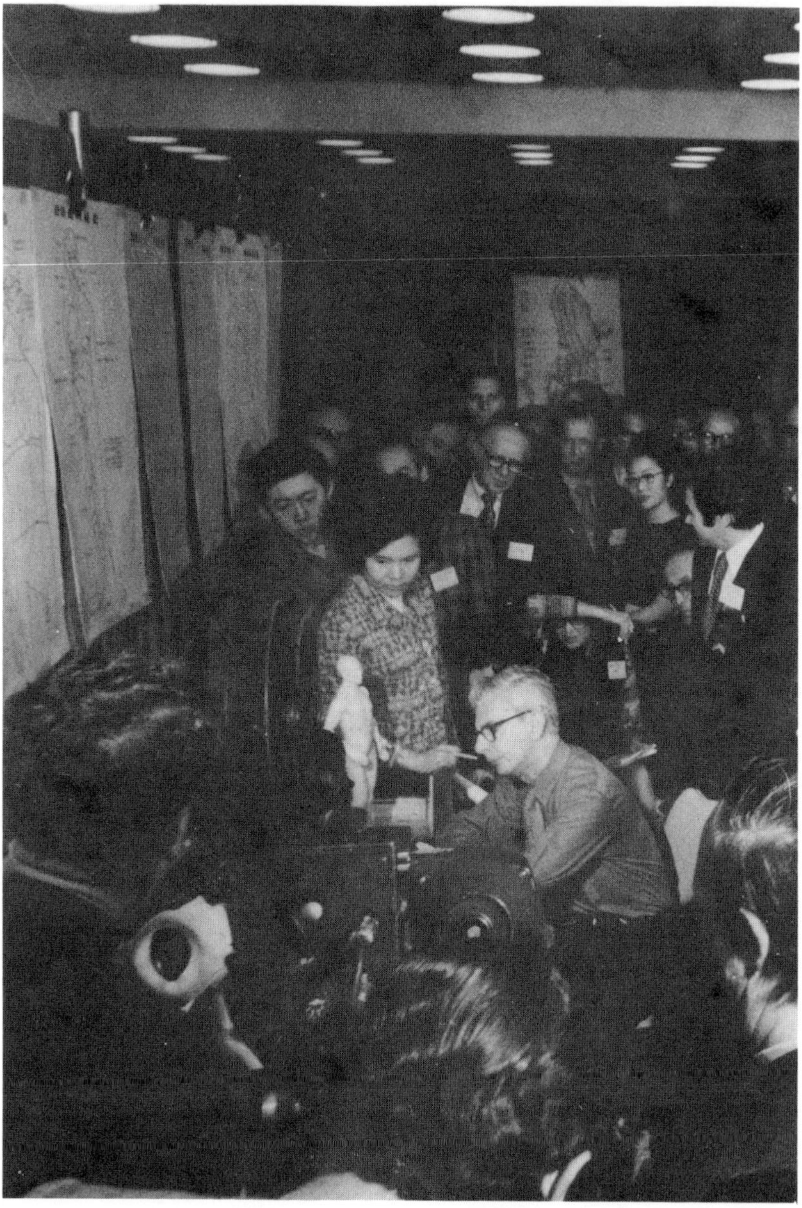

Scene at the first scientific acupuncture exhibition in the United States: the New York State Society of Anesthesiologists' Annual Meeting, December 14, 1971. The author won a Special Prize for his display on "Acupuncture in the United States."

HANDBOOK OF MEDICAL ACUPUNCTURE

Frank Z. Warren, M.D.

VNR
VAN NOSTRAND REINHOLD COMPANY
NEW YORK CINCINNATI ATLANTA DALLAS SAN FRANCISCO

Van Nostrand Reinhold Company Regional Offices:
New York Cincinnati Atlanta Dallas San Francisco

Van Nostrand Reinhold Company International Offices:
London Toronto Melbourne

Library of Congress Catalog Card Number: 76-3541
ISBN: 0-442-29198-1

Manufactured in the United States of America

Published by Van Nostrand Reinhold Company
450 West 33rd Street, New York, N.Y. 10001

Published simultaneously in Canada by Van Nostrand Reinhold Ltd.

15 14 13 12 11 10 9 8 7 6 5 4 3 2 1

Library of Congress Cataloging in Publication Date

Warren, Frank Z
Handbook of medical acupuncture.

Includes bibliographical references and index.
1. Acupuncture. I. Title. [DNLM: 1. Acupuncture.
WB369 W288h]
RM184.W37 615'.892 76-3541
ISBN 0-442-29198-1

To

Drs. Louis R. Orkin and Valentino D. B. Mazzia,
and to my daughters Rebecca and Kathy, who shared
the best and worst moments of my life.

F. Z. W.

PREFACE

This book is a beginning. It was first written in 1972 and has been revised three times prepublication in an effort to keep it up to date. Nevertheless, the field of acupuncture medicine has burgeoned so rapidly in the past three years as to render this task almost impossible. This volume represents the thought and practice, not only of myself, my staff and proximal colleagues, but also of other faculties from various sections of the country.

It could have been called *American Acupuncture* in an attempt to differentiate it from its Oriental predecessor, since it does not have the many advantages known to practitioners of the art in the Far East—namely, the concomitants of *moxa*, diet, massage, *Tei Chi*, deep breathing, and herbs (herbology almost always accompanies needling in China).

But, I trust, it also manages to escape the disadvantages—the dirty needles, the dogmatic empiricism, the overload of philosophy and propaganda, the factionalism and nationalism of different cliques—all of these have been sidestepped because they belong to the historical rather than the practical aspects of acupuncture.

This book is an entrance into a room filled with familiar objects, being seen for the first time in a new light. There is nothing startling about trigger points, electroanesthesia, electromyographic stimulation, transcutaneous or dorsal column stimulation, and other similar medical entities. We should not be recalcitrant about studying them, regardless of their local appellation, and should they fall into the catch-bag of acupuncture effects, they should not prejudice or congeal our thinking. We should, and shall, know them and encompass them unhesitantly. As Polonius says in *Hamlet*, addressing Laertes.

> Those days thou hast and their adoption tried
> Grapple them to thy soul with hoops of steel,
> But do not dull thy palm with entertainment
> Of each new watch'd unfledged remedy.

Acupuncture certainly is no unfledged remedy.

Frank Z. Warren, M.D.

New York City

MERIDIAN DESIGNATIONS	
Meridians	*Codes*
Lung	LU
Large Intestine	LI
Stomach	STO
Spleen	SPL
Heart	H
Small Intestine	SI
Urinary Bladder	B
Kidneys	K
Pericardium (Heart Constricter)	P
Tri-Heater	TH
Gall Bladder	GB
Liver	LV
Curious Meridian Point	CMP
Vessel of Conception	C
Governing Vessel	G

CONTENTS

HANDBOOK OF MEDICAL ACUPUNCTURE

FIFTY COMMONLY ASKED QUESTIONS ABOUT ACUPUNCTURE

In this first section I shall attempt to touch briefly on the questions which have been asked of me so many times in my lectures throughout the United States, Mexico, and Europe.

This type of question-and-answer section is usually relegated to the back of most volumes, but I have discovered that it seems to quickly and more effectively serve the reader's needs, and so I have moved it up front. It is to be hoped that by reading this section first, the student of acupuncture will approach the more detailed scientific sections with a broader outlook.

1. What is acupuncture?

Acupuncture derives from the Latin *acus* for "needle" and *pungere* for "puncture." This is the Western name given to one branch of treatment in Chinese medicine. It is not the name given to this method by the Chinese, who call it *chen chiu*, and who feel it is based on the *chinglo* or meridian theory of body physiology. It is important to note that acupuncture is only one facet of treatment in the Chinese approach to healing. It is hardly ever used alone, but always in combination with other branches of Chinese medicine, such as herbs, deep breathing, massage, diet, moxibustion, and other forms of therapy. These are combined to form a totally encompassing approach to the treatment of the human body and mind, which are never separated in Chinese medicine. The *chinglo* are invisible channels, connecting acupuncture points, through which courses the life force—*chi*, consisting of a balance between *Yin* and *Yang*, the positive and the negative. There are in all 12 paired and 2 unpaired *chinglo* and many other connecting, or conjoint, meridians.

2. What is moxibustion?

Moxibustion is another form of Chinese therapy related to acupuncture. The dried seed of a plant known as the mugwort (artemisia vulgaris) is affixed to the end of the acupuncture needles by means of a gluey matrix and ignited. The heat generated in this way travels along the length of the acupuncture needle deep into the tissue. It can be considered an early form of diathermy, without the electricity. In some cultures, moxibustion is practiced without acupuncture needles by igniting the substance directly on the surface of the skin and producing blisters, which sometimes result in the later formation of scars. I do not feel it will be of importance in the practice of acupuncture in the United States.

3. Is acupuncture in common usage throughout the world?

Acupuncture has been used for thousands of years in the Oriental cultures, and for decades on the European continent. Early references to acupuncture-like techniques go back as far as the Egyptian period, and references have been made in early acupuncture writings to dragons, which could have easily been an allusion to some remaining dinosaurs. At present, acupuncture is practiced by 150,000 licensed M.D.'s throughout the world; in China, where there are 800 million people; in Japan, where there are at least 15,000 M.D.'s practicing the Nakatani system; and in many other places, where lack of statistics prevents us from a definitive statement. It is only now being examined in the United States, Canada, Mexico, and South America. There are no available records of the African practice of acupuncture, although needles are used quite promiscuously in religious ceremonials. In India, Indonesia, and other parts of Asia, acupuncture is quite prevalent and practiced industriously by thousands of doctors.

4. How long should a United States doctor be required to study acupuncture?

A knowledge of Eastern acupuncture mythology, which requires two to five years in the schools of acupuncture found in the Orient, is not essential to the development and training of Western physicians.[1] For the most part, these schools insist on teaching the Chinese names, locations, and functions of the 365 to 1,000 acupuncture points on the body and multiple recipes, formulae, and applications in a large variety of conditions, the variation depending on which school of acupuncture one subscribes to. (See also Question 8.)[2] It seems fairly certain now that the meridian system is a philosophic, not a medical, entity. It has served its purpose well, but will soon be replaced by a sounder neurophysiologic theory. This makes the entire five-year concept and the rigorous training unnecessary. Also superfluous for our Western requirements is the arduous Chinese training required for taking and feeling the pulses in order to diagnose latent disease processes. Under controlled circumstances, this method does not seem to hold up. Since this technique requires a long and most intensive period of training, once this can be eliminated, the graduation of acupuncture-trained physicians can be accelerated. In China, when an accelerated program was mandatory, untrained girls were qualified as acupuncturists within three months.[3]

It is commonly believed here that in one year an anesthesiologist can learn enough basic acupuncture theory to allow him to acupuncture a patient with reasonable care, due caution, and diligence within our known ethical concepts. The presumption is that he has already prepared himself with some of the basic groundwork by having studied regional anesthesia, nerve blocks, and spinal anesthesia. In addition, he has an excellent background knowledge of various pain states and pain phenomena. Similarly, neurologists and neurophysiologists would have a head start in their study of acupuncture in that they too have been immersed in unraveling the neurophysiology of pain and painful conditions. The average family physician might require a little longer (approximately one and a half years). Rheumatologists and physiatrists have been practicing techniques in this country which closely resemble acupuncture. They should have no trouble adding acupuncture to their armamentarium.

A substantial amount of acupuncture can be learned in a solid, well-planned introductory course of 100 hours.

5. Is any knowledge of the meridian system of value?

As stated before briefly, the meridian system has great historic significance. It was developed as a working hypothesis before there was any true understanding of the physiology of the human body—before Harvey, Galen, Leeuwenhoek, Koch, Lister, and the others. It still has some function in that in average hands it teaches us where to stick needles into the body without inflicting catastrophic damage. However, as a working theory, it is inferior to the more modern neurophysiologic concepts today. Even the Chinese are abandoning it, as this quote from the *Peking Medical Review* will show.

> . . . it was found that about half of the known acupunctural points are located right over various nerves and the rest are within half a centimetre of one or another nerve. From this, the conclusion was

> drawn that acupuncture acts in fact on the nervous system and it is through a nerve that the stimulus produced by needling or applying a mild electric current is transmitted to a certain part or organ of the body where it effects a cure or brings about a state of analgesia. With this knowledge, additional acupunctural points have been located along the nervous system and they are not necessarily found on any of the *ching* described hitherto. By following the nervous system, medical workers have been able to pinpoint spots which are even more effective for anaesthesia than points formerly known.

As a system of geographical body notation, however, the meridian designation of acupuncture points is superb.

6. How precise are the locations of the meridians?

This question has been indirectly answered above. If one supports the meridian theory, then their locations are fairly precise, because there are always 12 paired and 2 unpaired meridians which course along the body, passing well-recognized landmarks, regardless of whether the patient is tall or slim, old or young. However, even the work of Professor Kim Bong Han, which purports to offer strong histologic substantiation of the anatomic presence of these meridians, has not convinced the Western community that there is any such thing as a meridian, and therefore the specificity of their locations cannot be corroborated.

7. How reliable are the relationships of the meridians to specific symptoms and ailments?

Since the meridian theory is not reliable, their relationships to symptoms and ailments are not reliable. It is important to note that this applies to meridians only and not to acupuncture points, which do have a certain specificity. However, even this is subject to individual and nationalistic variations.

8. How many acupuncture points are there?

The number of acupuncture points depends on which school the student attended and which books he has read. Originally there were 365 points, a number bearing a remarkable resemblance to the number of days in the year. Later, 500 more points were recognized. Later still, secret acupuncture points were discovered by various groups, cults, and acupuncture families, raising the total to over 1,000. Very recently, a group of new points was discovered in and around the ear, and other points on the nose and feet. Later, in the process of developing acupuncture anesthesia, all but a few points were abandoned. The Ryodoraku system has changed and reduced the number of points to a minimum. Neurophysiologists investigating acupuncture are working with groups of points which number from 40 to 80. Some of these coincide with acupuncture points and some do not. To answer the question of how many acupuncture points there are becomes a highly individualized process, depending on background, experience, state of education of the individual, and so forth.

9. How many of these points are commonly used by the professional acupuncturist?

A "professional acupuncturist" is usually defined as someone trained in the Orient whose basic working theory of acupuncture fits into the philosophic concept of Yin-Yang and who subscribes religiously to the meridian theory. In the average treatment, they employ between three to a dozen acupuncture points if they are not using electricity. Some of the more advanced acupuncturists, who have learned to employ electrical methods or needle-twirling, use fewer points. Combinations of points are used until the one most successful is discovered, mostly by empirical methods. More than one treatment is almost always obligatory; the points are changed, substituted, and new combinations of the known points developed for that specific individual and his specific complaint. Purists and "professionals" will deny this, but nevertheless that is the basis for their methodology.

10. How necessary is it that patients be acupunctured precisely at the acupuncture points?

Purists from the Orient insist that since acupuncture points are only a fraction of an inch wide, best results can be achieved only when the points are acupunctured *exactly*. Some primitive non-controlled tests have been submitted to show that this is so—that when a patient is acupunctured at an area a few millimeters to the side of the known acupuncture points, the desired effect is not achieved. In our experience, this is not so. When there is a known acupuncture point, going too far off to the side will achieve a result different from what is expected, but not any less effective. Furthermore, injecting a chemical analgesic such as procaine at the acupuncture site will frequently nullify the effect of that point, but the amount that need be injected is decidedly more than would be necessary just for the anesthetization of the tiny area that acupuncturists feel the point occupies. There are groups who feel that there is no such thing as an acupuncture point, but rather that there are points on the body at which a somato-visceral reflex can be instigated; or, conversely, that a viscera can give rise to a sensitized area on the skin. These phenomena, which have been known to us for years, are all part of the acupuncture panorama. In the ancient Orient, phenomena were explained solely on the basis of meridians, but we are developing a more consistent neurophysiologic basis.

11. What is the value of the "tobiscope" or "punctoscope" point-locators?

In some research centers these have been thought of as electronic toys, developed as part of the mystique of acupuncture. Other investigators swear by them. Suffice it to say that in their present state of development they are highly suspect, since the acupuncture points that they demonstrate move from day to day in the same individual; are changed by the addition of a drop of saline (which should enhance their capability); are affected by heat, cold, touch, pressure, and sweating. Scientifically, these variables make the findings of the instrument questionable. Our impression is that they may, from time to time, demonstrate the location of points where there is an increase in electromagnetic or ionic activity, but since this is caused by so many factors in the living body, it would seem unscientific to call the point at which this occurs an acupuncture point.

12. If point-locators are not too accurate, why are they so popular?

Point-locators, which look scientific and make satisfying noises—beeping and lighting up whenever a supposed acupuncture point is stimulated—satisfy both the doctor and the patient in a rather insubstantial scientific arena. Presumably it makes the chore of finding acupuncture points much simpler, thereby reducing the necessity for five years of study in order to locate the points.

Actually, its results are discountable, except perhaps in the auricle, where ear acupuncture points seem somewhat more constant.

13. What is the difference between tonification and sedation, using acupuncture needles?

Both terms refer to individual techniques of the introduction of the needle into the skin and the eventual effect on the patient and the "*chi*." Much is made of the angle of introduction, the motions of the fingers, and the depth to which the needle penetrates. Presumably, by varying these considerations, the meridian can be tonified, "hyped-up," excited (since it has been found to be deficient in "life energy"); or sedated, quieted down, depressed (if it has too much "life-energy"). Just another chapter in the mystical poetry of Yin-Yang. A discernible difference can be achieved if the needle is merely inserted, or if it is twirled, or if it is stimulated by a vibrator, or if it is stimulated electronically. And certainly the depth to which the needle enters the human body is extremely important, since in many cases it remains in the skin or reaches subcutaneous fat or muscle or even bone and synovial surface (as is suspected by many physicians). It is possible that dextro-rotation or laevo-rotation may be related to setting up opposing electrical fields in the tissue, but no studies have been done thus far.

14. What types of acupuncture needles are there?

Just as in the case of how many acupuncture points there are, so do we find a wide variation in the types of acupuncture needles. There are several flourishing schools of acupuncture, and each professes that its needles are the best. The Chinese, the Koreans, the Japanese, the Taiwanese, the Indians, the Germans, the Italians, and the French all have extremely dogmatic ideas concerning their needles. Most bizarre of all is the French idea that gold and silver needles are therapeutically more effective. The modern stainless steel acupuncture needle has come a long way from the bone and flint splinters of antiquity. It consists of a 32-gauge shaft and a handle which varies in shape and in size from country to country but which predominantly is meant to insure a firm grip and the capability of twirling without losing control. Materials such as copper or iron should never be used for needles, since with the addition of electricity they will polarize and deposit corrosive metallic elements deep within the tissues, producing burns. Needles vary in length from a half inch up to eight inches, depending on which function they have. In some special cases, they have been clumped in clusters to produce a dermal stimulation needle, called "plum blossom." Some needles, also called acupuncture needles, are enormous in size and are used for blood-letting, but this procedure is not our concern in this monograph.

15. What are the dangers of inserting acupuncture needles into the skin, and do you sterilize the needles?

Obviously, for the record, all needles which are inserted into the human skin should be sterilized thoroughly. In actual practice, few Chinese acupuncturists do more than swab the skin lightly with some astringent. Frequently they forget to do even that. Surprisingly enough, few localized abscesses are seen. A great deal depends on the condition of the skin before acupuncture, which obviously relates to the hygiene of the person. The Department of Health of the City of New York has records on a number of abscesses that have been observed where moxibustion is the modality, since burned tissue forms a good breeding ground for bacteria. In the hands of expert practitioners, it would appear that no more localized problems occur with acupuncture than with hypodermic needles, sterilized or not. A disposable needle would be the scientific ideal, since the cost of acupuncture needles is high. The best needles are made of stainless steel and can be sterilized and reused. Attention has been brought to the fact that a hypodermic needle punches out a core of tissue, carrying it inward, and would be more inclined to cause an infection, whereas the ultra-fine acupuncture needle insinuates its way through the layers, carrying very few cells from the surface with it. This could be corroborated by histologic studies.

16. What is the incidence of hepatitis caused by acupuncture needles?

Millions of acupuncture treatments have been performed, but since no statistics have been kept, all that can be said is that to the best of our knowledge, no hepatitis epidemic has ever been started as a result of acupuncture. This is startling, considering the promiscuous use of acupuncture in countries such as China, Japan, and India, where medical acupuncturists frequently use the same needle from patient to patient with scant prophylactic care other than a quick wipe. No doubt individual cases may have occurred without documentation. However, in this country, there are no verified cases of hepatitis initiated by acupuncture needles, although we have seen a good many allocated to our own Western techniques.

17. How long are the needles left in once they have been inserted?

Ordinarily, in classical Chinese acupuncture, needles are left in for a period of five to ten minutes. Occasionally they may be kept in longer; and in some instances, where the acupuncturist was treating a recalcitrant pain state, they have been left in overnight and even for a period of several days. In these cases, special precautions are employed, such as cutting the needle, discarding the handle, and including the remainder in a protective bandage, thereby allowing the patient freedom of movement. In Japan, small metal balls are sometimes used as reinforcements of the needle. These, too, are worked into the bandage over the acupuncture points.

Since the advent of electricity as an augmentation to acupuncture, overnight or two-day treatments seem to have diminished. Twirling and electrification seem to provide adequate carry-over stimulation, adequate for the period between treatments in the patient's course of therapy. Stimulation by the electrical machines can vary from five minutes to thirty minutes per treatment. In the case of prolonged surgical operations, they obviously must be continued throughout the course of the operation, which can take up to six or seven hours in the case of pneumonectomies and other chest operations. There seem to be no side effects regardless of the length of stimulation, but precautions regarding burns should be maintained.

18. How long does the analgesia last?

The analgesia or pain-blocking effects produced by acupuncture vary widely, from a few minutes to a few days, and in extraordinary instances may extend for months and years. The duration is independent of the amount of stimulation. For example, there is one well-publicized American case of a 48-year-old lady with shoulder problems who was acupunctured once and whose analgesia lasted for almost a year. As in other phenomena of pain, explanations for startling results are not always handy.

19. What is the advantage of twisting or electrifying the needles?

Both of these techniques are relatively new, having first begun in the Orient in the 1950s. We are still accumulating information with regard to this question, but it appears to us now that both twirling and electrification provide a superior stimulation, producing analgesia and symptom relief for long periods with minimal application. It is important to note that the two methods are not interchangeable. The electronic machine puts out a rather complicated wave form which cannot be stimulated merely by twisting or twirling the needle. It also avoids the fatigue factor in long surgical cases and obviates the necessity of several acupuncturists per patient in the operating room or the treatment annex. It allows much shorter periods of stimulation to effect much longer periods of analgesia, and affords us a measure of standardization and control not possible with the old-fashioned classical methods.

20. What is the most effective wave form of the electronic machine?

The original 626 machine, which is manufactured in the People's Republic of China, puts out a rather complicated wave form which consists of a biased square wave and several types of stimulation with varying band widths, densities, and Hertz. The most effective frequency found on this machine was between 80 and 100 Hertz, with 30 to 50 microamperes, and 25 to 35 volts. It produced trains of electronic impulses described in Chapter XI.

21. What does the patient feel when the needle is inserted, and is there any indication as to when the needle should be taken out?

There are subjective feelings influencing the length of each treatment. The arbitrary application of a time period applies more to electrical treatment. When the needle is first inserted, the patient gets a sensation called "the needle feeling," a flushing or tingling, which extends down the length of the extremity or over the area involved. Not achieving this "needle feeling" does not necessarily mean that the needle is not at the proper place, but it is a useful guide when it happens.

The Chinese emphasize that in order to be effective, the needle must hit the right spot to produce *t'chi* (getting the spirit), which consists of four sensations, namely, *suan* (soreness), *chung* (swelling), *ch'ung* (heaviness), and *ma* (numbness). These sensations correspond to the sensations resulting from a mild stimulation of the peripheral nerve and/or a tetany of the adjacent muscle.

As far as subjective feeling is concerned, the wide variations from patient to patient have taught us to ignore subjective statements and confine ourselves to the monitoring of the patient's physical signs. These undergo distinct changes—vasoconstriction, normal tonicity, vasodilatation, and others. These changes can be demonstrated and are discussed in greater detail in Chapter VI. As far as termination of treatment, the Chinese believe that when a feeling of heaviness and dullness has been reached, the treatment can be terminated. In fact, some Chinese theorists have described it as being difficult to pull the needle out, and they consider this the termination point. Others insist that at this point the treatment has only begun and more time is needed.

22. Are there special retrieval techniques for the acupuncture needle?

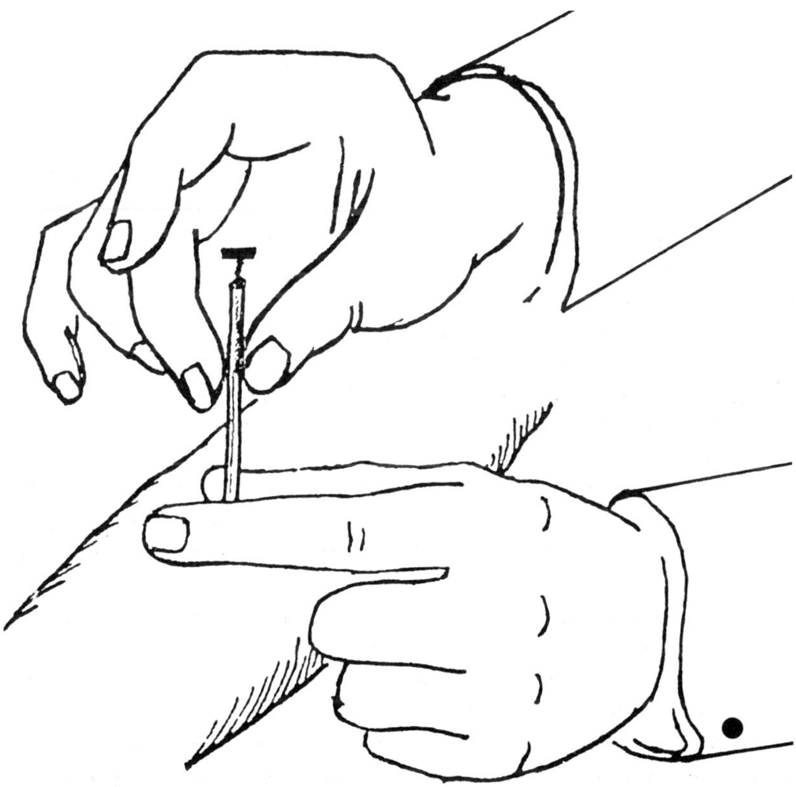

In Western medicine, one of the predominating fears is that a needle will break off in the patient's body and that the physician will be unable to retrieve it. This idea has carried over into acupuncture. Because the needles are much thinner and longer, and because the whole *gestalt* of acupuncture is unfamiliar, the fear seems to have reached epidemic proportions. Let me reassure my colleagues, if an acupuncture needle is well made, it will rarely break. Most of them are well manufactured of stainless steel and are flexible enough to bend but not to break. It is most difficult for even the strongest pair of hands to break this needle *in vitro*, and there is no reason to presume that the quiescent tissue of the average patient is any stronger. Techniques for insertion are more important than retrieval techniques. Experienced acupuncturists will find no difficulty in inserting even the very long, fine needles. Neophytes may discover, to their happy amazement, that an "introducer" (a sort of sleeve) will be of great assistance in handling the problem of needle insertion. *(Photo Slide)*

23. What are the advantages and disadvantages of acupuncture analgesia?

The answer to this question must be prefaced by the statement that we are not proposing acupuncture anesthesia as a substitute for the Western practice of anesthesia. As an adjunct it has superlative applications, but we are not ready yet to throw away our anesthesia machines.

Some of the advantages are obvious. Any modality which will slow the acceleration of drug usage is a preferred entity. Acupuncture anesthesia not only offers this possibility with anesthetic agents per se, but also the possibility of reduced usage of premedicants and post-operative analgesics. Another advantage is that in expert hands it is an innocuous procedure. Although there are effects on the heart, blood pressure, pulse, etc., no results have been observed that can be considered deleterious. The voluntary cooperation of the patient can be obtained during the operation. In some operations, such as pneumonectomy or thyroidectomy, this cooperation helps the surgeon, particularly by the avoidance of damage to important nerves, through talking to the conscious patient. Because it is non-chemical, it avoids the necessity of eliminating toxic materials, and thus the post-operative recovery period is extremely brief or completely eliminated. Furthermore, the analgesia produced in the operating room frequently extends through this post-operative period. In an emergency, it can be performed by personnel less highly trained than the anesthesiologist. It does away with the usual elaborate preparations and equipment required for surgery. It offers another agent of choice, particularly in poor-risk cases. The amount and number of endotracheal intubations can be reduced, perhaps even eliminated.

Some of the disadvantages are that it is cloaked in myth and mysticism, difficult to dispel, and therefore prone to be practiced by quack practitioners who profess themselves experts but who turn out to be less than adequate. It is difficult to standardize, and controlled experiments are difficult to set up and evaluate. In the surgical amphitheater, when it does not work, it can cause acute embarrassment to the personnel and stress and tension to the patient.

Very little experimental work is available at this time, although many plans are in progress. For the next few years this condition cannot be expected to improve, and it can be attributed to the fact that the only suitable subject for the study of pain in humans is a human being. Pain is a complex entity, different in animals, and difficult to measure in either case.

24. What acupuncture points have been used to produce analgesia for major surgery in this country?

Change of opinion regarding the location and number of acupuncture points is taking place even as this monograph is being written. Originally, such classical acupuncture points as LI 4, STO 36, B 2, P 6, TH 7 have been the most popular points of stimulation for producing analgesia. Several years ago the Chinese stated that all the acupuncture points necessary for analgesia anywhere in the body could be located in and around the pinna of the ear, and since then they have reduced the 200-odd points so indicated to about three. If acupuncture pain theory is valid, these three points, when stimulated, should produce analgesia throughout the body. Should their stimulation prove inadequate, they can be augmented by stimulation of the additional points along the appropriate nerves. These are seen in the following illustration:

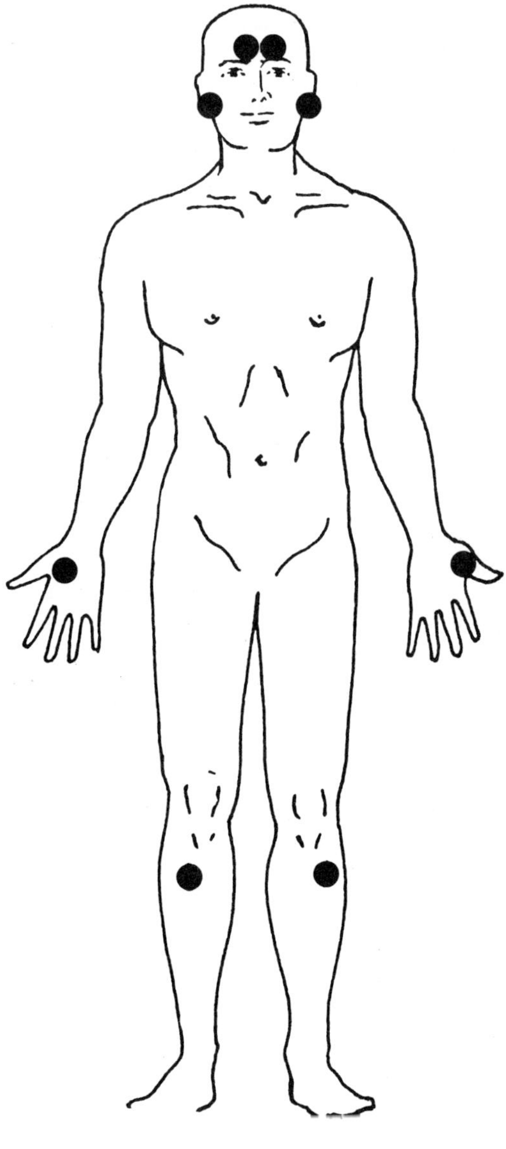

25. What are the points used in minor surgery?

Where minor surgery involves the lower abdomen, the *tsu sanli* (STO 36) points can be used. Where it involves surgery above the abdomen, *hoku* (LI 4) and ear and eye points can be used.

Another technique is to surround the operative site with electrified needles imbedded in the skin. This method is used in plastic surgery, small fibromata, sebaceous cysts, salivary incisions, dental work, and other small operative sites. In caesarian sections, the classical obstetrical points are augmented by two eight-inch-long needles implanted in the rectus abdominus on each side along the line of incision. In dental surgery, the classical *hoku* points (bilaterally) may be augmented by an ear point on the affected side. Recently in China, particularly in children, analgesia has been accomplished without needles by intense pressure on acupuncture points in the face, cheek, and ear, for a period of five to ten minutes immediately preceding the extraction. However, in extensive dental work, such as full-mouth repairs or multiple extractions, the standard techniques and well-known points should be used.

26. How long does it take to develop analgesia using these electronic techniques?

The average length of induction is 15 to 20 minutes, although some operators have required only five to eight minutes for dental operations, and others have required 30 minutes and more for abdominal operations. If this seems too cumbersome for everyday practice, one must remember that in the early days of ether anesthesia this was approximately the time it took to produce a surgical level of anesthesia. Scheduling the preparation of the patient in a side room by an assistant while the preceding operation is carried on will allow for this induction time. The optimum method for handling the time required for the development of analgesia with acupuncture depends as much on the facility of the acupuncturist as does the anesthetic on the anesthesiologist.

27. What is meant by pulse diagnosis?

Pulse diagnosis is a method used by practitioners of traditional Chinese acupuncture to determine the nature of the imbalance in the "Yin-Yang." It is similar to Western medicine in that in both cases the radial pulses are the ones felt. However, it differs in that they claim twelve pulses can be identified, six on each wrist, by feeling for three superficially and three deeply. Here again, the skill of the practitioner allows him to distinguish fine differences in these twelve pulses and make a diagnosis. In actual practice, it has been found that using this system, different acupuncturists will diagnose different ailments in the same patient. Since this is one of the facets of acupuncture which takes so long to learn, and since it is so random in its results, it seems foolish to dedicate a great deal of time to studying and learning pulse diagnosis. Should it prove of future value, a device with electronic sensors and a readout similar to the EKG tracing could easily be developed to make this method of diagnosis less speculative and individualistic. Why adjacent portions of the same radial artery should feel different is still inexplicable at this time.

28. What is the Ryodoraku system of diagnosis and treatment?

This is a system of acupuncture which claims to pre-date the Chinese acupuncture anesthesia development by ten years. It has 15,000 adherents in Japan, and in its application and practice appears to be more simplified than the Chinese, depending on the autonomic nervous system. Although it is still reminiscent of certain basic aspects of the meridian theory, it remains important enough for further study. (See Chapter V.)

29. What types of ailments are treated most frequently by acupuncture?

Tic doloreux
Dental conditions
Torticollis
Hiccup
Cervical herpes
Causalgia
Raynaud's disease
Acute vascular occlusion
Cerebral accidents
Herpes zoster
Postoperative intercostal pain
Herpes
TBC laryngitis
Headache
Limitation of shoulder and arm
Angina
Frostbite
Hyperhydrosis
Bronchial asthma

Paroxysmal tachycardia
Fractured ribs
Idiopathic chest pain
Fractures of the costal cartilage
Thrombophlebitis
Arterial occlusion
Hirschprung's disease
Chronic ulcers
Sciatica
Lower back pain
Minor fractures, manipulations, mobilization
Postoperative atelectasis
Postoperative scars
Phlebothrombosis
Chronic peripheral vascular disease
Epidydimitis and salpingitis
Coccydinia
Gangrene of the extremities

29a. We must now list the common specific ailments treated most frequently by nerve blocks:

Gangrene of the extremities
Coccydinia
Epidydimitis and salpingitis
Chronic peripheral vascular disease
Phlebothrombosis
Postoperative scars
Postoperative atelectasis
Idiopathic chest pain
Fractured ribs
Paroxysmal tachycardia
Bronchial asthma
Hyperhydrosis
Frostbite
Angina
Limitation of shoulder and arm
Headache
TBC laryngitis
Herpes
Minor fractures, manipulations, mobilization
Lower back pain

Sciatica
Chronic ulcers
Hirschprung's disease
Arterial occlusion
Thrombophlebitis
Fractures of the costal cartilage
Postoperative intercostal pain
Herpes zoster
Cerebral accidents
Acute vascular occlusion
Raynaud's disease
Causalgia
Cervical herpes
Hiccup
Torticollis
Dental conditions
Tic doloreux

Please take note that both lists are identical. For instructive purposes, I have merely changed their sequence in order to make my point. Others are listed in the pathophysiology section.

30. What are the comparative results of the effectiveness of these two methods of treatment (nerve block v. acupuncture)?

Approximately the same in many cases. In fact, it is to be considered that the placebo factor in nerve-block treatment is very high when compared with acupuncture and hypnosis. Some authorities feel there is no placebo acupuncture point, all points having some effect.

31. Is acupuncture just another form of hypnosis?

This question is too important to be handled summarily. In brief, the statistics seem to imply that acupuncture, while it includes hypnotic components, goes far beyond the capabilities of hypnosis both in treatment and in surgery. (See Chapter VII).

32. What are the contraindications to acupuncture?

It is almost a foregone conclusion that if a Chinese acupuncturist is asked if acupuncture can help this or that condition, he will almost automatically say yes. In China, not surprisingly, acupuncture is used for almost everything. This includes the infectious diseases, glaucoma, hearing difficulties, psychiatric disorders, and many other pathologic disturbances where one would never expect it to be used and where pain is not involved. This lack of discrimination in the use of acupuncture must not influence our practice. Antibiotics are faster than acupuncture, particularly where there is a specific organism. Psychotropic drugs work better than acupuncture in acute psychotic states. Other areas, where a choice of Western v. Oriental pharmacology can be made, should be explored, but one must not listen to the repeated remonstrations of the acupuncturists that acupuncture is good for everything.

Acupuncture is not used during pregnancy, nor is it commonly used as an analgesic in the Chinese delivery room in the normal birth process. In obstetrical pathology, it is employed, and, as we have seen, it has been used extensively in caesarian sections. Acupuncture is not recommended as a therapy for carcinoma, although there should be some value in its application for the relief of the pain.

This next idea must be emphasized: *There are acupuncture points which can cause death,* although most acupuncturists smilingly insist that acupuncture cannot hurt you. When we stop to consider that many acupuncture points coincide with military-arts points and evaluate the function of these points—which is to maim or kill—we can easily dispute the flippant claims of acupuncture's innocuousness. There are also a number of points which are known to cause syncope and general collapse. These will not be published here. In general, therefore, although acupuncture has few contraindications, a fundamental knowledge of anatomy, physiology, and pathology, and a thorough history are essential to its practice.

33. What ailments now treated with acupuncture by Western practitioners provide hope for maximum success in the future?

Thus far, although only a scattering of results has been reported in the United States, acupuncture seems to offer promise in the areas of painful arthridites, psychosomatic diseases, and as an auxiliary for anesthetics in the operating room. Post-operative pain and distention also seems a good candidate for investigation. Deafness is not a fertile area for exploration. Dentistry is.

34. What ailments treated with acupuncture by Western practitioners seem to offer no success?

Cancer, tuberculosis, and degenerative nerve diseases such as amyotrophic lateral sclerosis, multiple sclerosis, and Pick's Disease, are the areas in which acupuncture would seem to offer the least promising results. Likewise, deafness is not yielding the high degree of satisfactory results that we anticipated.

35. What are the acupuncture points commonly used for obstetrical analgesia?

These points are not known, because in China the delivery of a baby is considered a normal process, one which does not require analgesia, as opposed to methods applied to pathologic conditions. Thus, there are no points recommended for obstetrical delivery in the Oriental text. However, in this country, where the mother-to-be feels constrained to enact an opera of pain and suffering in order to give birth (the basis of which has never been fully explained), certain acupuncture points will provide analgesic relief. The recipe for these points will vary according to the patient and the acupuncturist, but commonly used sites are the ones used for dysmenorrhea and ovarian malfunction. Caesarean sections are more practical, using points we will list in the appendix.

36. Do acupuncture points have any value?

Before answering this question it is necessary to define much more clearly what an acupuncture point is. Acupuncture points, fixed, classically oriented, specific for specific diseases, combined or individual, do not really exist. Nonetheless, it is known that there are points or loci scattered on the surface of the human body which have characteristics unlike the rest of the skin surface. They do not fall into straight lines, as meridian theorists would like us to believe. Electrical resistance is diminished at these points; spectographic characteristics are changed; palpation appears to indicate a looser, less-dense tissue consistency; electrical activity registers higher on a galvanometer; and the insertion of a needle, or pressure at these points, will produce local and sometimes central systemic changes when applied vigorously and for long enough periods. Neurophysiologists commonly recognize forty to sixty such points, and work with them for transcutaneous stimulation. When, in a diseased state, they have been accompanied by inflammation and soreness, they have been described as trigger points. They are not constant, varying from individual to individual and within the same individual. In general, these points can be described as places where a needle can be inserted to an average depth of one-half to two inches without extraordinary damage—pneumothorax, pericardial abrasion, rupture of a viscus, or penetration of a large blood vessel. Careless insertion at these points can cause excessive trauma and even death, certainly no different than in Western medicine. A knowledge of classical Chinese acupuncture points acts as a reminder of these dangerous loci. Since their location and distribution varies from person to person and from race to race, to memorize their names in Chinese, Japanese, or any other language can only be considered an interesting intellectual exercise. If one is interested in teaching, all the various major points can be remembered by their numerical meridian number rather than by their Chinese name. Meridian numbers (e.g., Large Intestine 4) are at least recognized world-wide and are understood universally. Teaching acupuncture in antique languages can only serve to create a mystique, the basis for cult practice.

37. Is there a typical number of treatments for the relief of a given ailment?

In the best hands, acupuncture is dose-related just like any other medication, particularly when the application of electrical current is added to the acupuncture treatment. The question is reminiscent of the query regarding the number of shock treatments necessary for a disturbed psychotic. Treatments are given until the patient has either shown improvement or definitely convinced the practitioner that this form of therapy will not help. It is customarily necessary to try various combinations and types of application for treatments. One-treatment remissions are rare, but do occur where the psychosomatic factor is high. It is interesting to note that although the Chinese claim great success with acupuncture in all categories of human pathology, they are well aware of a good percentage of failure. In acupuncture anesthesia, where the patient's reactions to the knife allow results to be more easily determined, they claim a modest 90 per cent success.

38. Which conditions can acupuncture cure completely?

There are *no* conditions that acupuncture can cure completely, any more than there are any conditions that Western medications *cure*. In this respect, both systems of treatment are similar. They are aware that they do not cure anything but rather that they restore the homeostatic balance and allow *Nature* to cure the pathologic disturbance. Too many Western practitioners do not know, for instance, that penicillin is a bacteriostatic. It does not kill, but immobilizes, so that the immunologic body forces can then overpower the invader. In acupuncture, some internal relationship is affected, brought about by the changes produced in the blood pressure, pulse, sedimentation rate, enzyme balance, hormonal output, and psychic reaction, allowing the body to overcome the pathologic process.

39. Can I, as a registered M.D. practicing medicine, practice acupuncture?

In the very near future, this question will be academic. At this juncture, the consensus is that acupuncture can only be practiced within an approved protocol cleared by a Human Research Committee affiliated with a medical center. In New York State, where the Acupuncture Committee of Dr. Jackson Riddle and Dr. Pascual Sanchez has performed superlatively, a requirement of 100 hours of training has been added.

40. Does this mean that if you are not on the faculty of a medical center, you cannot practice acupuncture?

If acupuncture, pure and simple, is what you practice, then the answer is yes, that's what it means. However, if, as in the case of anesthesiologists, neurologists, physiologists, rheumatologists, psychiatrists, and other doctors in related categories, you are involved in the practice of medicine which includes pain control, and if, in the presence of intractable pain which has not responded to conventional methods of treatment, you are faced with a decision of performing the insertion of a needle with or without the barrel of novocaine customarily attached to it, and if your patient has been fully informed of what you are doing and has signed a paper to that effect, then by virtue of your license to practice you may perform that procedure. What you must avoid doing is to say that you are practicing acupuncture. You may call it a nerve block based on neurophysiologic work, or any other euphemism. You need not call it anything. As long as you inform the patient of what you are doing, what the consequences may be, what the side effects may be, or that there may be unknown side effects, and if you have a good relationship with that patient, no harm can come to you for the insertion of that needle. This is not be interpreted as an encouragement to immediately get hold of some acupuncture needles and make pincushions of your patients. There must be concrete indications that you have exhausted all conventional methods and that you are a reasonably cautious and careful doctor; and the informed consent must include your patient's knowledge that by not giving her a syringe full of novocaine you are performing an experimental procedure, odd as it seems. These are the inconsistencies of acupuncture practice as they now exist. A much fuller discussion is found in a later chapter.

41. Is acupuncture likely to be accepted in the United States?

It is hoped that acupuncture will prove itself out in the United States, as it did in France. In 1930, when it was introduced there by Soulie de Morant, it was greeted with the same wave of skepticism, but today it is an accepted form of medical practice, and only M.D.'s can use it.

42. Should unlicensed practitioners who are expert acupuncturists be allowed to practice acupuncture?

This question could be rephrased to state: "Should unlicensed practitioners who are expert acupuncturists be allowed to practice medicine?" In any number of major states, acupuncture has been adjudged the practice of medicine, and until these barriers are lifted, only M.D.'s in medical center settings can legally practice acupuncture. Recently, in California, M.D.-supervised qualified personnel have also been allowed to perform acupuncture as part of a research protocol, and there are a number of psychologists who are actively treating patients within this framework. The New York State formula also includes a provision for them. In Nevada, they may practice alone, which in our opinion constitutes a dangerous health hazard.*

*Unfortunately, New York State has recently passed a law which will allow nonphysicians to practice.

43. Now that we know all about acupuncture, how does it work?

No one really knows how acupuncture works, any more than anyone knows how aspirin works or how anesthetics work. And who said we know all about acupuncture other than headstrong local journalists? Even the Chinese have just begun their research.

44. Why is this so?

This is so because acupuncture is intimately interwoven with the phenomenon of pain, a much-discussed and hotly-debated subject for many years, and an entity for which we have as yet no clear-cut understanding. (See Chapter VII.)

45. What is the Government attitude towards acupuncture?

At an acupuncture meeting that was held on March 2, 1973, convened by the National Institute of General Medical Science in Washington, the Government representative displayed less skepticism than ever before and an eagerness to start the research phase of acupuncture. More than eighty scientists were convened, and ideas and information presented and exchanged. Interest in the subject was evidenced from universities all over the country, and undoubtedly many of them will be awarded research grants in the very near future. All seemed to agree that there was something worth looking into, and even the one or two die-hard skeptics had some related area which they felt could be investigated with productive results.

46. Is the AMA against acupuncture?

The American Medical Association has displayed a totally open-minded attitude towards acupuncture. They have published an extraordinary authoritative report of what was seen in China by Dr. E. Grey Dimond, Provost for Health Sciences in Kansas University Medical Center, and have followed this up with pictures, one or two scientific reports, and a definite encouragement to researchers in the field. One or two AMA "mavericks" mistakenly oriented towards the drug profession have said some unscientific things, but otherwise they have been comparatively fair.

47. What is the attitude of the pharmaceutical companies towards acupuncture?

In the present state of the science, acupuncture poses no serious threat to the revenues of the pharmaceutical companies. In fact, several companies have been instrumental in supporting lectures on acupuncture, and a number of them went so far as to distribute acupuncture needles and literature, although the feeling was it was more to get attention than to support the field. In the operating room, acupuncture anesthesia will not replace chemical anesthesia except in certain selected and poor-risk cases. It could easily become a welcome addition to the armamentarium of the anesthesiologist in situations where the anesthetic history precludes conventional methods. Ugly rumors continue to circulate regarding a slush fund designed to help prosecute the first acupuncture malpractice suit. No verification of this rumor can be discovered.

48. Where can one send patients for treatment?

At this point, it is not advisable to prescribe acupuncture treatment for any patient until all other standard medical prescriptions have been exhausted. Acupuncture is not a disease, nor is it a category; it is a treatment. In fact, in the Chinese tradition, it is a treatment meant to be combined with other treatments. When a lay person sends in a patient for acupuncture, he is prescribing a treatment—perhaps the wrong treatment, and perhaps thereby misdirecting attention to an experimental modality when regulation methods might be adequate. One does not send patients anywhere for acupuncture. One sends patients to a physician, who might then feel that acupuncture may be pertinent and useful. They allow the physician his prerogative of prescribing what he thinks is the proper medication, instead of ordering the medication before the diagnosis has been made. If these foregoing statements seem pedagogic, I must apologize, because I know intractable pain is a terrible driver of people. When a patient is in severe pain, he wants help, not hair-splitting opinions, and this wordy explanation cannot alleviate that pain—better to have the address of a competent acupuncture practitioner.

The National Acupuncture Research Society publishes the only authoritative directory of acupuncture clinics and practitioners.

49. How effective is acupuncture in dentistry?

Because of the circumscribed pathology found in dental practice, acupuncture is infinitely more applicable than in medical practice. In fact, it is my feeling that doctors of dentistry will be in the forefront in the establishment of acupuncture in this country. A great deal of the research now being planned involves using the teeth as a standard of measurement for pain, since accepted methods of pain measurement are extremely subjective, ineffective, and subject to false interpretation.

50. What are the fiscal aspects of acupuncture?

Because of the enormous press and medical interest in acupuncture, unscrupulous people, both in and out of the profession, have profited from the agonizing situation of patients suffering from intractable pain of a variety of origins. A pain-driven patient, desperate for relief, will pay anything to anybody who can produce that relief. This is the atmosphere in which quack practitioners flourish. A relatively large group of non-medical acupuncture graduates from Hong Kong and Taiwan has somehow made its way to these shores and has proceeded to treat desperately-ill patients without regard for either the diagnosis or the results. In some cases, licensed doctors have encouraged these non-professionals, and the fees, ranging from $25 to $100 per treatment, have amassed them a large bank account. Capitalizing on human pain is not only unethical and immoral but beyond comprehension and needs no further comment. One advantage of the seemingly restrictive law requiring that patients be treated in medical centers is that quite possibly there will be no fee. The deplorable fact is that in this country there are large numbers of patients in constant pain who have been abandoned by the medical profession, not because of neglect or incompetence, but merely because for most of them there is nothing more that can be done. It is to be hoped that in the acupuncture modality some relief can be found for them, and it is essential that while we are looking for it, they are not exploited. And it is even more essential that we hurry.

REFERENCES

1. *The Yellow Emperor's Classic of Internal Medicine (Huang Ti Nei Ching Su Wen)* circa 2696-2598 B.C., translated by Ilza Veith, Baltimore: Williams and Wilkins, 1949.
2. The Peking Acupunctural Anesthesia Cooperation and Coordinating Group, "Spots, Meridians and the Principle of Acupunctural Anesthesia," *Mung Chi*, No. 12, Nov. 1971.
3. The Peking Acupunctural Anesthesia Cooperation and Coordinating Group, "The Principle of Acupunctural Anesthesia," *Peking Medical Review*, pp. 17-20, Feb. 1972.
4. Ilza Veith, "Acupuncture Therapy—Past and Present," *J.A.M.A.*, May 12, 1968, 134-140.
5. Patrick D. Wall, "Cord Cells Responding to Touch, Damage, and Temperature of Skin," *J. Neurophysiol.* 23, 1960, 197-210.
6. W.F. Collins et al, "Relation of Peripheral Nerve Fiber Size and Sensation in Man," *Arch. Neurol.* 3, 1960, 381-385.
7. Michael Patkin, "Measurement of Tenderness with the Description of a Simple Instrument," *Med. J. of Australia*, March 28, 1970, 670-672.
8. William E. Hunt and James L. O'Leary, "Form of Thalamic Response Evoked by Peripheral Nerve Stimulation," *J. Comp. Neurol.* 97, 1952, 491-514.
9. Karl O. Von Hagen, "Chronic Intolerable Pain," *J. Amer. Med. Assoc.*, 165:7, Oct. 19, 1957.
10. William F. Collins and Clark T. Randt, "Midbrain Evoked Responses Relating to Peripheral Unmyelinated or 'C' Fibers in Cat," *J. Neurol.*, 23, 1959, 7-53.
11. John J. Bonica, "Acupuncture Anesthesia in the People's Republic of China," *J.A.M.A.*, 229:10, Sept. 2, 1974, 1317-1325.
12. Philip R. Trommer and Milton B. Gellman, "Trigger Point Syndrome," *Rheumatism*, July, 1952.
13. Philip M. Toyama and Michimasa Nishizawa, "The Traditional Oriental Medicine and Acupuncture Therapy," *J. Mississippi State Med. Assoc.*, 14:11, Nov., 1973, 488-495.
14. Alan Van Poznak, "Advances in Electrosleep and Electroanesthesia During the Past Decade," *Clinical Anesthesia*, 502-520.
15. Ronald Melzack, "Phantom Limb Pain," *Anesthesiology*, 33:4, 409-419, Oct., 1971.
16. "Suppression of a spinal and a cranial nerve reflex by vaginal or rectal probing in rats," *Brain Research*, 35, 1971, 231-235.
17. Alan Van Poznak, "Electrical Anesthesia," *Anesthesiology*, 24:1, Jan.-Feb. 1963.
18. C. Norman Shealy, et al, "Current Status of Dorsal Column Stimulation," A Synopsis of the Doral Column Study Group meeting, April, 1971.
19. Peking Acupunctural Anesthesia Co-ordinating Group, "The Principle of Acupunctural Anesthesia," *Peking Review*, Feb. 25, 1972, 17-20.
20. C. Norman Shealy, et al, "Electrical Inhibition of Pain by Stimulation of the Dorsal Columns, *Anesthesia and Analgesia*, 46:4, July-Aug., 1967, 489-491.

21. C. Norman Shealy, et al, "Electrical Inhibition of Pain: Experimental Evaluation," *Anesthesia and Analgesia,* 46:3, May-June, 1967, 299-305.
22. William H. Sweet and James G. Wepsic, "Treatment of Chronic Pain by Stimulation of Fibers of Primary Afferent Neuron," Trans. *Am. Neurol. Assoc.,* 93, 1968, 103-107.
23. Wall and Sweet, "Temporary Abolition of Pain in Man," *Science* 155, 2967, 108-109.
24. Pan L. Man and Calvin H. Chen, "Acupuncture Anesthesia: A New Theory," Personal Communication.
25. Peking acupuncutral Anesthesia Cooperation and Coordination Unit, "Spots, Meridians, and the Principle of Acupunctural Anesthesia," *Hung-ch'i* (Red Flag), 12, Nov. 1, 1971, 79-87.
26. Sin-I Cheng, "Electric Activity of Nerves as a Foundation of Acupuncpuncture and Chinese Medicine," Private Communication, Nov. 1971.
27. Harold S. Saita, "Modern Scientific Medical Acupuncture," *J. AOA,* 72, March 1973, 685-696.
28. Henry Nemerof, "Clinical Experiences with Acupuncture," *J. AOA,* 71, June 1972, 866-873.
29. Henri Rathle, "Acupuncture in the Pain Syndrome," *J. Med. Assoc. State of Alabama,* 43:2, Aug. 1973, 87-91.
30. G. Weddell, *Annu. Rev. Psychol.,* 6:119, 1955.
31. Sinclair, D.C.: *Brain,* 78:584, 1955.
32. Livingston, W.K.: Pain mechanisms, New York, MacMillan, 1943.
33. Collins, W.F. and Randt, C.T.: Fiber size and organization of afferent pathway, *Arch. Neurol.* 5:202, 1961.
34. Shealy, C.N.: The physiological substrate of pain. *Headache,* 6:101-108, 1966.
35. Wall, P.D. and Sweet, W.H.: Temporary abolition of pain in man, *Science,* 155:108, 1967.
36. Sweet, W.H. and Wepsic, J.C.: Treatment of chronic pain by stimulation of fibers of primary afferent neuron. Trans. *Am. Neurol. Assoc.,* 93:103-107, 1968.
37. Shealy, C.N., Taslitz, N., Mortimer, J.T., and Becker, D.P.: Electrical inhibition of pain, experimental evaluation, *Anesthesia and Analgesia,* Current Researches, 46:229-305, 1967.
38. Shealy, C.N., Mortimer, J.T. and Reswick, J.B.: Electrical inhibition of pain by stimulation of the dorsal column. Preliminary Clinical Report, *Anesthesia and Analgesia,* Current Researches, 46:489-491, 1967.
39. Shealy, N.C., Mortimer, J.T. and Hagfors, N.R.: Dorsal column electroanalgesia, *J. Neurosurg.* 32:560, 1970.
40. Shealy, N.C., Adams, J., Brown, R., Clark K. and Hunt, W.: Current status of dorsal column stimulation, A synopsis of dorsal column study group meeting held in Dallas, Texas, April, 1971.
41. Lam Kin-Hung. Needling anesthesia, *Hong Kong,* Ping-Chun Publishing Co., p. 14, Sept. 1971.
42. New acupuncture believer: Nixon's doctor, *Medical World News,* p. 17-19, April, 1972.

CHAPTER I

TWENTY-FIVE ACUPUNCTURE POINTS MOST ESSENTIAL TO YOUR PRACTICE

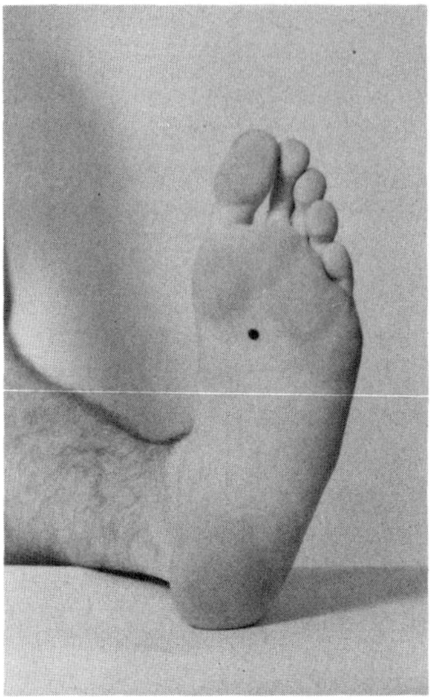

KIDNEY 1

One-third the distance from the center to the front of the planta surface, in the depression which is present when the foot is compressed laterally.

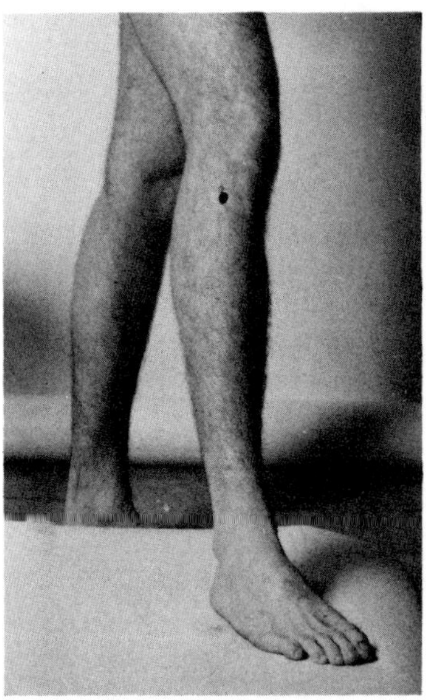

STOMACH 36

3 tsun (body inches) below the tuberosity of the tibia on the lateral side of the anterior tibial crest in the tibialis anterior muscle.

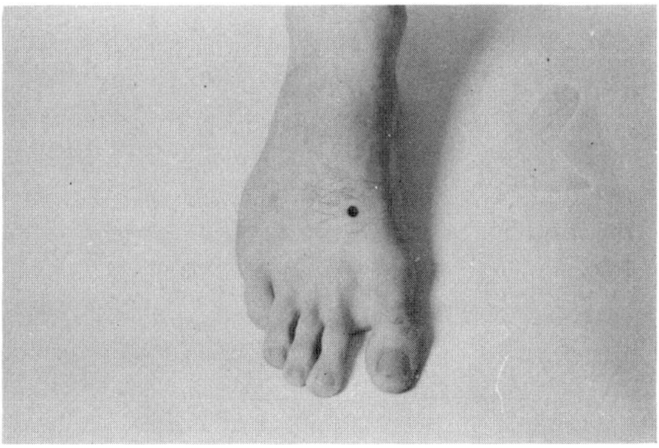

LIVER 3
Over the depression between the first and second metatarsal bones, approximately 2 tsun proximal to the web between the big toe and the second toe.

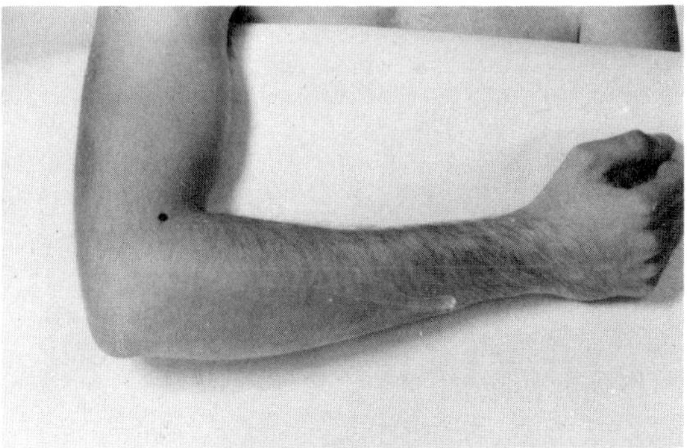

LARGE INTESTINE 11
At the lateral end of the elbow crease when the elbow is flexed.

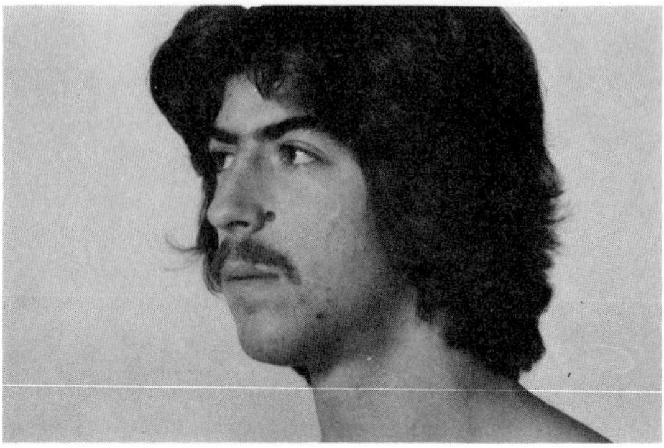

LARGE INTESTINE 20

0.5 tsun from the side of ala nasi, in the nasolabial sulcus.

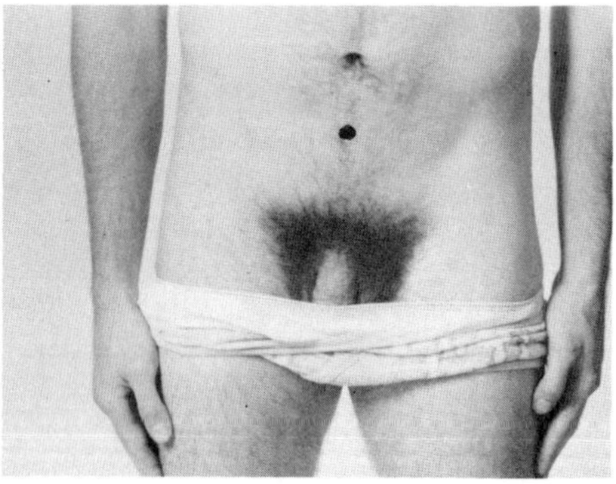

CONCEPTION VESSEL 4

3 tsun below the umbilicus.

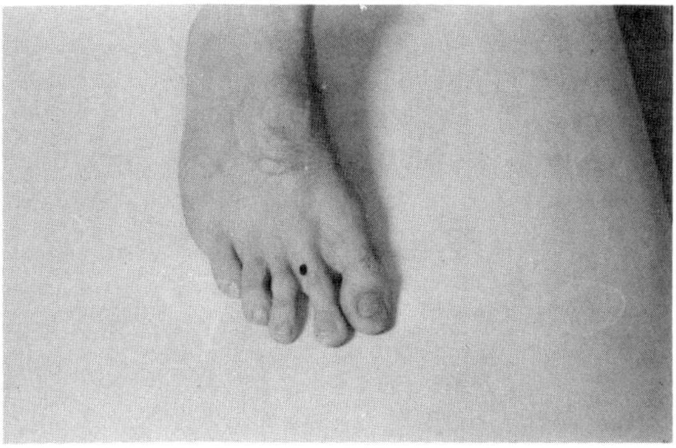

STOMACH 44
In the web between the second and third toes.

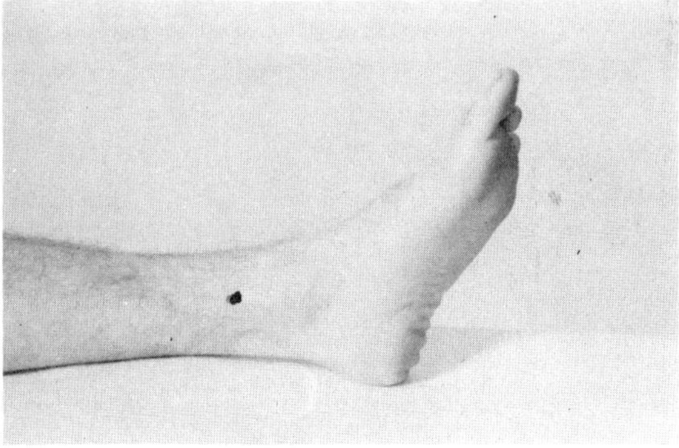

SPLEEN 6
3 tsun above the apex of the medial malleolus, behind the tibia.

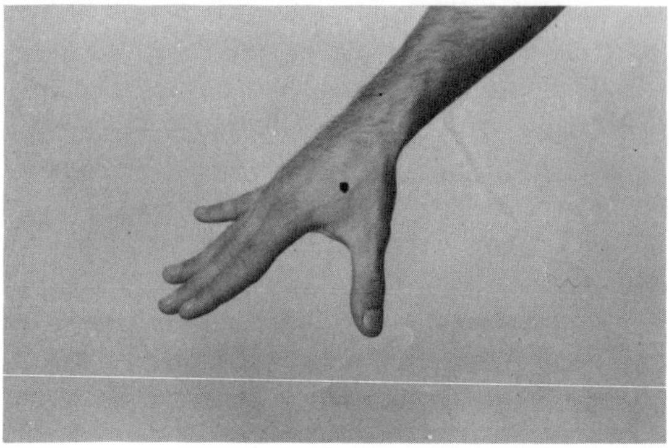

LARGE INTESTINE 4

On the dorsal surface of the hand, between the first and second metacarpals, on the protuberance of the muscle on the radial side in the middle of the metacarpus.

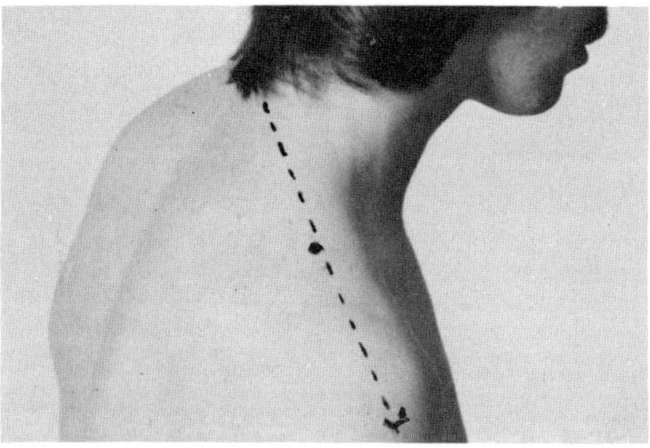

GALL BLADDER 21

On the hump of the shoulder, midway between C7 and the acromion.

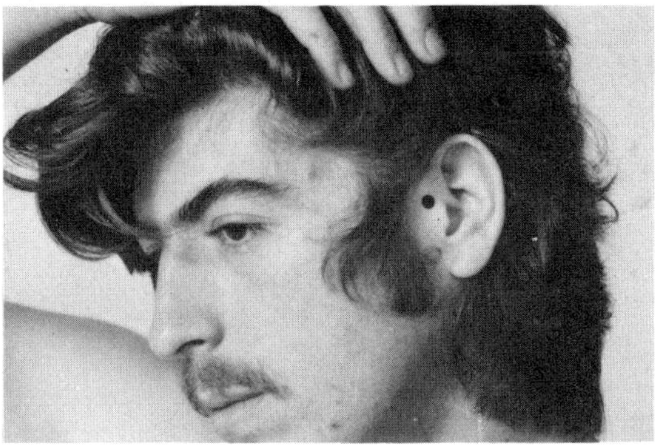

SMALL INTESTINE 19

Between the middle of the tragus and the mandibular joint, where a depression is formed when the mouth is opened.

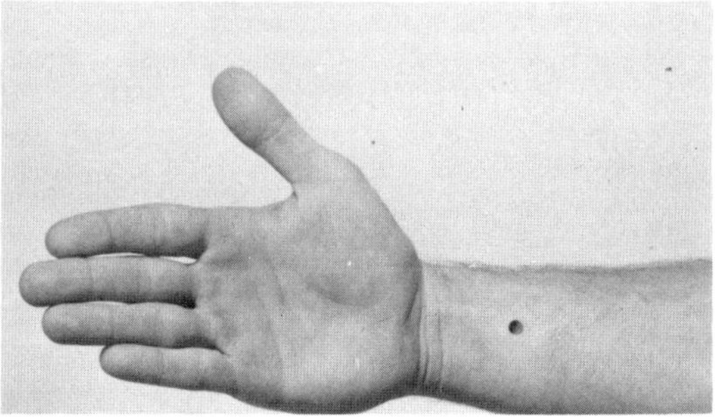

PERICARDIUM 6

2 tsun above wristfold between the two tendons of the palmaris longus muscle and flexor carpi radialis muscle.

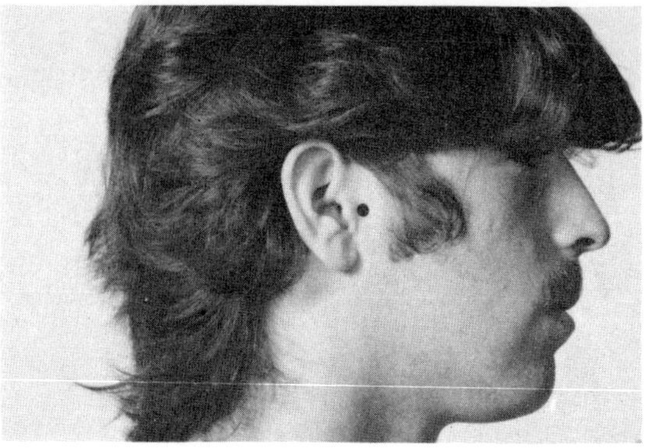

STOMACH 7

In the depression between the inferior border of the zygomatic arch and the mandibular notch.

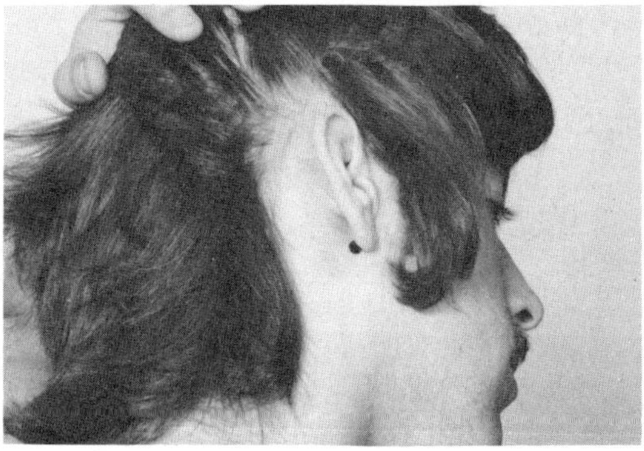

TRIPLE BURNER 17

Behind the lobule of the auricle, in the depression between the mastoid process and the mandible.

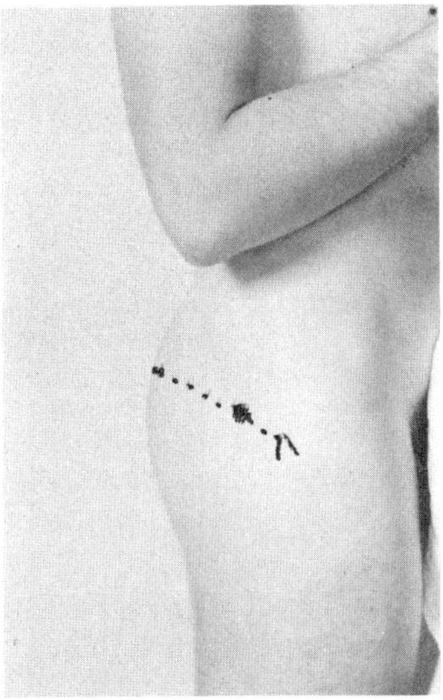

GALL BLADDER 30

On the postero-superior side of the greater trochanter, ⅓ the distance, posteriorly, from the greater trochanter to the sacral hiatus.

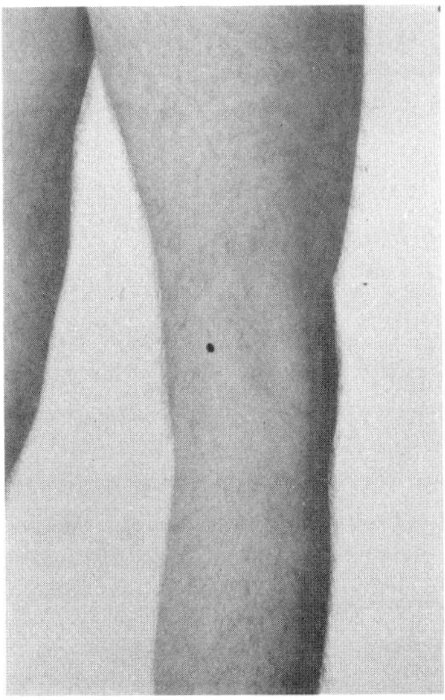

GALL BLADDER 40

(54 in some charts)

Right in the middle of the popliteal fossa.

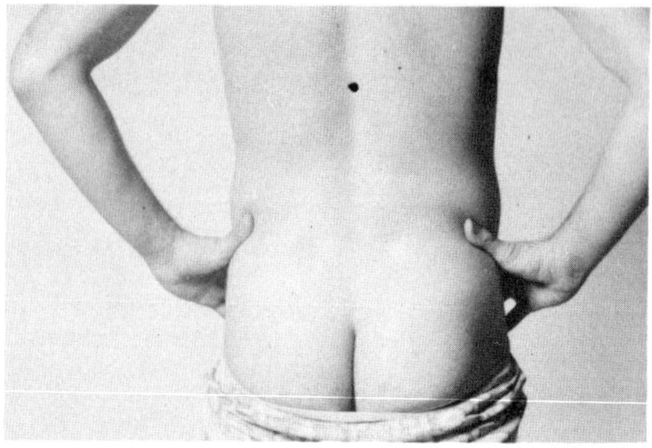

GOVERNING VESSEL 4

Below the spinous process of the 11th thoracic vertebra.

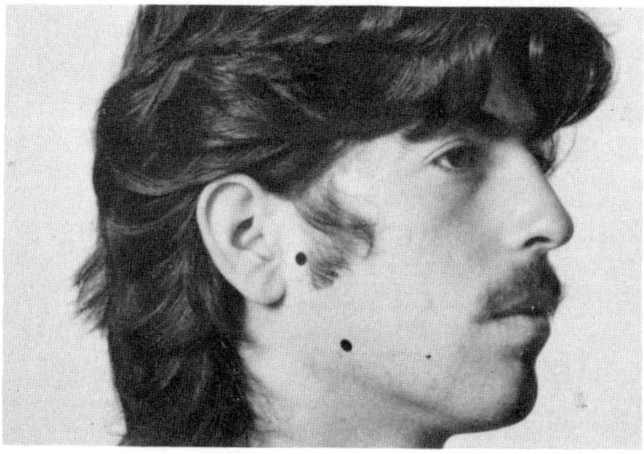

GALL BLADDER 2

On the posterior margin of the condyloid process of the mandible, in front of the insisura intertragicia, where a depression is formed when the mouth is wide open.

STOMACH 6

Over the masseteric muscle anterior to the angle of the mandible.

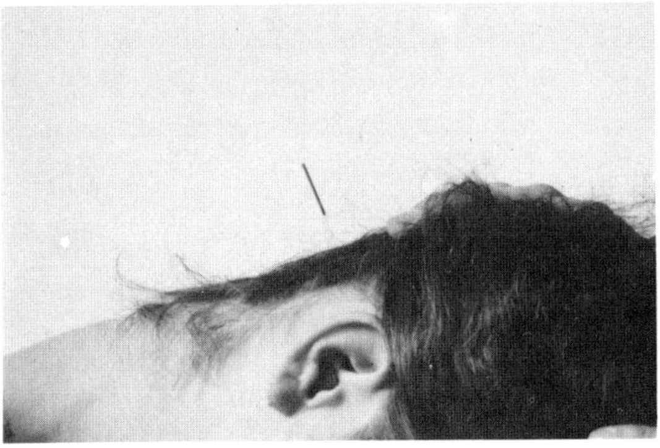

GALL BLADDER 20
Below the occipital bone, in the depression on the outer part of the trapezius muscle, on a level with Bladder 10.

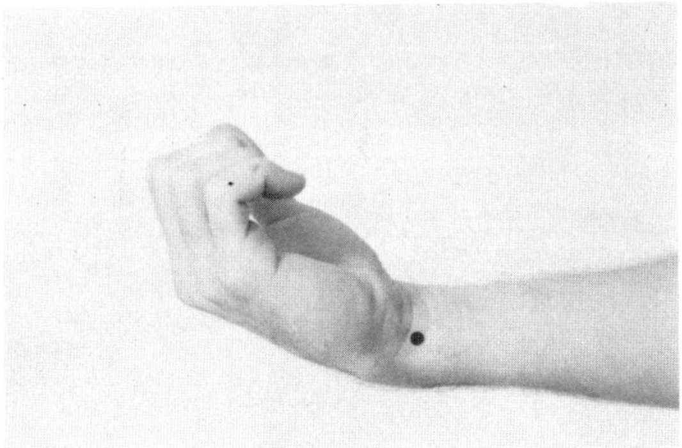

HEART 7
Along the most distal skin crease of the wrist on the ulnar side of the flexor carpi ulnaris muscle.

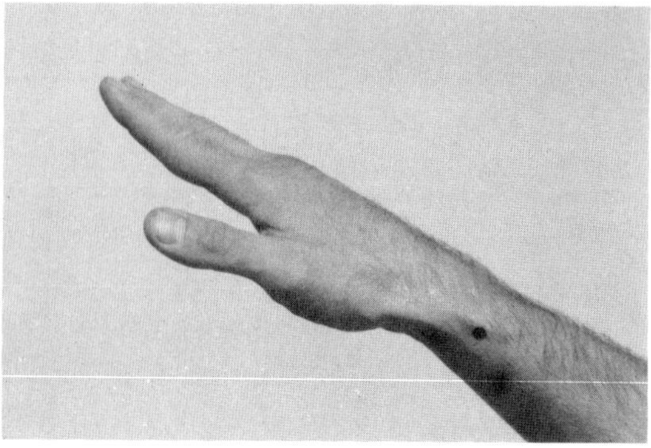

LUNG 7

1.5 tsun above the most distal skin crease of the wrist above the styloid process of the radius.

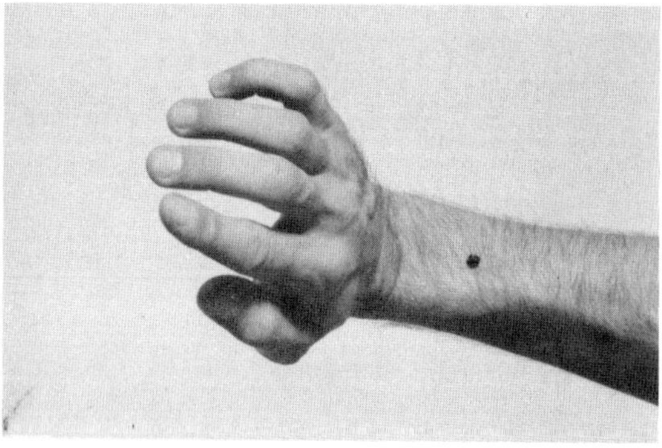

TRIPLE BURNER 6

3 tsun above skin crease on the back of the wrist, between the ulna and the radius.

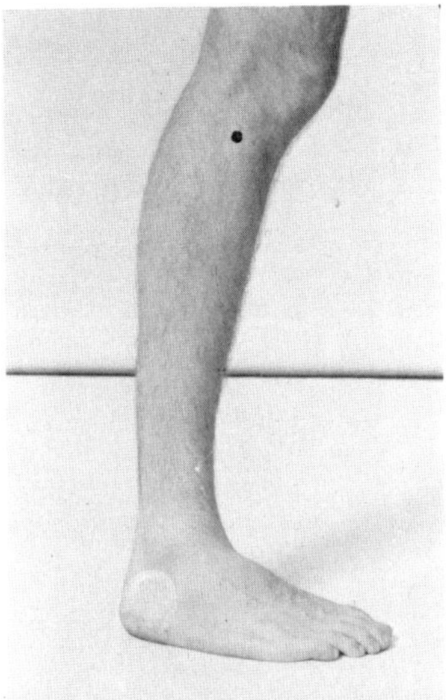

GALL BLADDER 34

On the anteroinferior part of the capitulum of the fibula, 2 tsun below the knee.

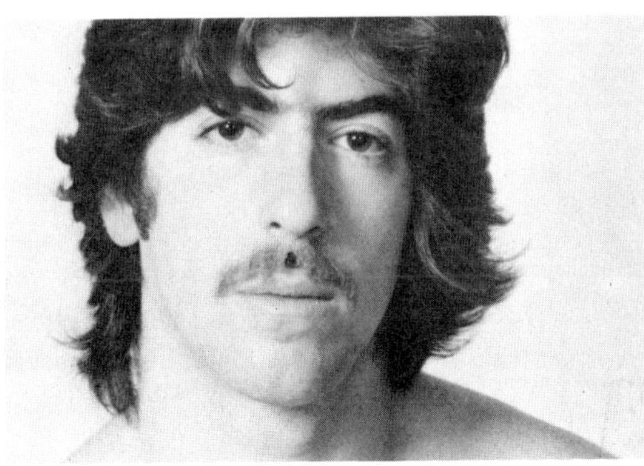

GOVERNING VESSEL 26

Just above the middle of the philtrum.

MAJOR THERAPEUTIC APPLICATIONS:

Stomach Meridian:

Pt. 6 Toothache; parotitis; facial nerve paralysis; trigeminal neuralgia; locked jaw.

Pt. 7 Toothache; deafness; tinnitus aurium; inflammation of the mandible; facial nerve paralysis.

Pt. 36 General tonification; gastritis; ulcer diseases; diarrhea; distended abdomen; constipation; indigestion; high blood pressure; anemia; hemiplegia; epilepsy; neurasthenia; insomnia.

Pt. 44 Stomachache; headache (frontal); toothache; tonsillitis; dysentery.

Large Intestine Meridian:

Pt. 4 Headache; toothache; rhinitis; swollen and painful oropharynx; deafness; eye disease; facial nerve paralysis; fever; upper limb joints pain; hemiplegia; neurasthenia.

Pt. 11 Arthralgia in upper limb; paralysis; "wind rash"; hemiplegia; shoulder and back pain; swollen and painful oropharynx; high blood pressure; goiters.

Pt. 20 Occlusion of nose; rhinitis; nasosinusitis; facial nerve paralysis.

Spleen Meridian:

Pt. 6 Irregular menstruation; dysmenorrhea; menorrhagia; nocturnal urination; impotence; frequent micturition; abdominal pain; diarrhea; indigestion; neurasthenia; hemiplegia; premature ejaculation; insomnia; weak uterine contraction during labor.

Pericardium, Heart Constrictor, Envelope of Heart Circulation-Sex Meridian:

Pt. 6 Thoracodynia and costalgia; stomach pain; insomnia; palpitation; hiccough; nausea; vomiting; asthma; swollen and painful oropharynx; hysteria; epilepsy; chest surgery.

Gall Bladder Meridian:

Pt. 2 Deafness; tinnitus; otitis media; toothache; facial nerve paralysis; mandibular arthritis.

Pt. 20 Headache; eye diseases; rhinitis; common cold; apoplexy; hemiplegia; deafness; tinnitus.

Pt. 21 Shoulder and back pain; neck pain; difficulty in raising the arm; mastitis; hyperthyreosis; functional metorrhagia.

Pt. 30 Lumbar pain and pain in the legs; sciatica; paralysis and paresis of the lower limbs.

Pt. 34 Knee joint pain; sciatica; hemiplegia; costalgia; trauma of the joint.

Triple-Burner Triheative Triple Warmer Meridian:

Pt. 5 Upper arm joints pain; paralysis; hemiplegia; parotitis; deafness; tinnitis; neck pain.

Pt. 17 Deafness; tinnitis; facial nerve paralysis.

Heart Meridian:

Pt. 7 Nervousness; forgetfulness; insomnia; palpitation of the heart; hysteria.

Lung Meridian:

Pt. 7 Headache; stiff and painful neck; cough; asthma; facial nerve paralysis.

Liver Meridian:

Pt. 3 Headache; fainting spell; vertex pain; high blood pressure; menorrhagia; amenorrhea; mastitis.

Kidney Meridian:

Pt. 1 Vertex pain; infantile convulsions; unconsciousness; heatstroke; cerebral hemorrhage; hysteria; epilepsy.

Small Intestine Meridian:

Pt. 19 Deafness; tinnitus; otitis media; otitis externa.

Bladder Meridian:

Pt. 54 or 40 Lower back pain; leg pain; sciatica; hemiplegia.

Governing Vessel Meridian:

Pt. 4 Lumbar pains; enuresis; impotence; leukorrhea; endometritis; parametritis; headache; deafness; tinnitus; asthma.

Pt. 26 Shock; collapse; heatstroke; unconsciousness; hysteria; epilepsy; acute lumbar sprains.

Conception Vessel:

Pt. 4 Abdominal pain; diarrhea; dysentery; irregular menstruation; dysmenorrhea; leukorrhagia; impotence; enuresis; dysuria; urethrodynia.

CHAPTER II

ANATOMY OF A DERMAL PUNCTURE POINT

In the beginning we must classify the attitudes of the physicians who evaluate acupuncture, for this evaluation is of extreme importance in comparing intercultural results. It has often been said that a man is down on what he is not up on. Physicians approach acupuncture in different ways, depending on their state of maturity and their degree of sophistication. First they smile. Why do they smile? Well, it's a funny technique—the needles, the spots, the mystery, Chinese names sounding like a menu.

The next stage of development is the feeling that acupuncture is a Chinese Communist political ploy. China has nothing to sell except acupuncture and ping-pong, and the Sinophiles are at it again.

The third phase is that acupuncture is pure hypnosis. By now, there is a lot of accumulated evidence in this country to prove that there is no statistical relationship between the degree of hypnotizability and the therapeutic response to acupuncture. As we all know, there is an element of hypnosis in all therapeutic situations that exists in acupuncture as well.

The next phase is that there is something to it after all and maybe we ought to take a serious look at it, which is the stage which most of us are at today.

The fifth and final phase, I hope, will be its application in therapeutic practice, which is yet to come.

Which brings us back to the definition and description—the anatomy, if you will—of an acupuncture point. Because of the prejudice and confusion we have all been enduring, first what is required here is a new terminology. I suggest the term "dermal puncture point" so that we can once and for all unlimber our minds from the congealed thinking which accompanies the mention of the word acupuncture.

So many half-baked definitions of acupuncture points have been given that it seems unnecessary to add another, so let me repeat what I have often said before: that there are no acupuncture points. There are points on the skin, dermal points, which, when stimulated, will produce internal reactions. And there are internal derangements which will produce alarm, pressure or trigger points on the skin. And there are also points where are found neurologic bundles of mixed somatic fibers or large circulatory vessels whose walls are richly supplied with networks of autonomic fibers. I believe that any of these can carry an acupuncture message and deliver an acupuncture-like effect.

Before the advent of acupuncture in the United States we were fully aware of a great many phenomena which can be considered part of the acupuncture panorama. For example, some of the acupuncture points—particularly those in the back—are not unlike trigger points. If we remember properly, trigger points have been described in this country by such investigators as Trommer, Travell and Gelman, who referred to a structure in the skin, which, under sympathetic control, normally acts as an arterial-venous-capillary shunt, for the purpose of maintaining the homeostatic state, general blood pressure, circulation to the digits, and local and general body temperature. This structure may undergo benign tumefaction and cause a definitely recognizable painful condition, say Drs. Downs and Love. By speculation, therefore, trigger points appear to be hyperesthetic regions existing as painful nerve endings in the skin, subcutaneous tissue areas, fascia, muscle, or blood vessels. That they exist in the superficial skin layers is shown by the relief that is often afforded by the simple measure of intracutaneous procaine block. These bodies may correspond to the intracutaneous nodules palpated by acupuncturists. They may be the glomus body of Masson-Popoff. Considering the physiology of pain, an anatomically unrelated neuro-muscular-vascular disturbance may be explained on the basis of James Evans' hypothesis of causalgia. Trigger points have been discussed by Travell as the cause of disability in many conditions resembling and aggravating sacroiliac disease, the angina pectoris syndrome, and other afflictions having painful points which do not ordinarily fit into any known definitive nervous, skeletal, and muscular syndrome. In addition to these painful nodules, the surrounding skin appears to be hypersensitive to other stimuli, such as heat and cold, and without doubt, to the puncture of a sharp needle. For the most part, these intracutaneous points act exactly like acupuncture points in that they show manifestations of underlying disease.

The clinical conditions which must be considered here are migraine, Horton's Syndrome, hypertensive encephalopathy, rupture of the nuclear pulposus—the disc syndrome—peripheral vascular disease, sciatica, joint disease, herniation of subfascial fat, lumbosacral or sacroiliac disease, neuritis, gout, causalgia, myositis, and fibrositis—precisely the ones which yield the most gratifying results when treated by acupuncture.

According to Toyama, an American physician, acupuncture points and the Head's areas of referred pain seem to correspond. Sir Henry Head postulated that cutaneous pain felt in visceral diseases is located in areas where sensory nerves enter the spinal cord at the same segments which supply nerves to the viscera concerned. Some of the well-known acupuncture points which have a known effect on a specific organ, particularly those on the back, are in the appropriate Head dermatome. For example, Bladder 14—the thirteenth point on the bladder meridian, which is a point on the back situated just medially to the upper angle of the scapula—is said to influence the lungs when it is stimulated; and it falls within the known dermatomes of the lung, which are T 2 to T 9. Bladder 23—a point in the small of the back that is stated to influence the kidney—likewise falls within the proper dermatomes: Thoracic 9 to Lumbar 3. In fact, a chart is found in Mann's books that shows a fairly close relationship between the names and numbers of the acupuncture points, the organs influenced by stimulating these acupuncture points, and the dermatomes of that particular organ as we know it.

All of these points—whether called trigger points, acupuncture points, or alarm points—undoubtedly have the ability of causing fluctuations in a galvanometer held nearby, provided conditions of sweating, atmospheric pressure, and electronic phenomena are standardized. We can choose to call them acupuncture or even dermal puncture points in the future, or we can choose to keep their acupuncture designation such as Kidney 24 or Spleen 13. It is merely a geographic convenience to help us locate the exact point on the body to which we are referring. Like a music notation on paper, it provides a common vocabulary which transcends language barriers. It is my impression that the ancient Chinese did just that. But here in the United States, in 1975, to call them acupuncture points and to ascribe to them all the catalogue of effects brings into play the whole spectrum of superstition, Yin-Yang, and Oriental philosophy, whose screen we are trying to pierce to get at the why and how of needling phenomenology. So let us proceed.

How many dermal puncture points are there? The classical Chinese figure of 365 to 1,000 can be increased if we include secret acupuncture points discussed only in clandestine Chinese family meetings. They can be diminished in actual clinical practice to no more than 40 or 50. Some investigators, such as C. Norman Shealy and his associates, claim that 40 or 50 areas satisfy fully their requirements for stimulating all parts of the body. They use needles sometimes, but most times resort to transcutaneous stimulation. (See Chapter III.)

One Philadelphia investigator, Dr. Matsumoto, has reduced the number of functional puncture points to around 30. Dr. Nakatani, a Japanese investigator, practicing a Japanese form of acupuncture called Ryodoraku, has also simplified the number of points and the system of classifying them. More importantly, the classical acupuncture points are now being abandoned, even by the Chinese. They no longer call them "acupuncture points" and now refer to them as "loci." As recently as 1972 they have stated that all the body loci required for stimulation throughout the organism are replicated in the pinna, and the NARS chart* will represent their interpretation of the more important areas. Advanced investigators have claimed that two or three points are all that are required for total body analgesia, such as in the major operations. We have all seen their remarkable films. Study of these films reveals that in most cases one needle stimulation was the predominant anesthetic. We are working to find out how this was accomplished.

What are the characteristics of these dermal puncture points? They have been said to be of looser consistency, but this certainly does not apply in the pinna. They have been claimed to have diminished resistance to electrical current. The resistance between a large indifferent electrode and a point electrode held against acupuncture points was 20,000 to 80,000 ohms with a direct current of 20 to 100 microamperes. Their electrical potential varies, while that of normal skin is fairly consistent: there are 5-7 cycles of variation with an amplitude of 0.1 millivolts during a period of 3 to 6 seconds. Sometimes there is no period of inactivity, while sometimes it lasts several minutes. These alterations in potential were only noted at acupuncture points, and, to a lesser extent, in their immediate neighborhood. These electrical potentials are influenced by the physiological processes of the body and also by certain emotional states. What is suggested here is that they *are* the physiologic processes and the measurement variations are reflecting *normal* activity. A drop of saline anywhere on the skin will

*An acupuncture chart published by the National Acupuncture Research Society showing the most important ear acupuncture points.

affect the resistance to electrical current by virtue of its higher conductivity and will seemingly create acupuncture points or make them move over. Conceivably these puncture points may be the result of an increased concentration of sweat glands. Possibly they are near concentrations of myoneural end-organs. It has been claimed that puncture points contain also an unusually high amount of Pacinian and Krause corpuscles and other sensory end-organs; but this again poses a contradiction, because if so many end-organs and so many sweat glands are clumped together, shouldn't the result be a denser cutaneous consistency rather than a looser, as has been reported? It has also been reported that the spectroscopic absorption, particularly at the ultra-violet and infra-red ends of the spectrum, has been peculiar to these points; but there again, body oils, salts, and unnatural daily constituents of the sweat may be responsible. There is evidence that ingestion of extraordinarily high amounts of foods whose end-products are excreted through the skin can change these absorption properties considerably. And always, none of this applies to the ear, where the Chinese claim all points are represented.

So what are we talking about? What is the anatomy of an acupuncture point? Is there any? Are we talking about something tangible, a structure or an electronic response to an instrument, or a geographical landmark? I say the latter. We must not continue cultish obeisance to an ancient idea, established before there was knowledge of bony or surface anatomy. If we do, our progress in research will be impeded, but it will not hold back advances in China because they have already junked the ancient ideas. In 1972 they decided that:

> . . . it was found that about half of the known acupunctural points are located right over various nerves and the rest are within half a centimetre of one or another nerve. From this, the conclusion was drawn that acupuncture acts in fact on the nervous system and it is through a nerve that the stimulus produced by needling or applying a mild electric current is transmitted to a certain part or organ of the body where it effects a cure or brings about a state of analgesia. With this knowledge, additional acupunctural points have been located along the nervous system and they are not necessarily found on any of the *ching* described hitherto. By following the nervous system, medical workers have been able to pinpoint spots which are even more effective for anaesthesia than points formerly known.

So that for the rest of our work and studies in acupuncture, I suggest that when we hear reference to acupuncture points, let us not think of them as circumscribed anatomical structures—but rather as convenient reference points. And, of course, the permutation of these acupuncture points into the well-publicized neatly arranged rows called meridians is, to my mind, another convenient landmark meant to convey a teaching idea, rather than a positively-identified anatomical structure to be considered in the same category as vessels and nerves.

At one time it was thought that pain was a specific, such as touch and temperature, and that it followed transmission pathways which could be clearly outlined. Today most neurophysiologists have discarded this and, supported by investigation, feel pain is a psychophysiologic experience modified by many things. Similarly, acupuncture is really a *conglomerate* consisting not of points and meridians but of many transmission methods and pathways, some identified and some not too clearly marked out. Further, acupuncture points can be understood if we refer to them as dermal puncture effector points. Modern writers feel that they may be nodules or areas of concentrated chemical energy related to adenosone tri-phosphate—the same ATP which is ubiquitous in energy messages throughout the rest of the body.* We may scoff at the idea of "energy," but nevertheless the human body is teeming with chemico-electrical fields at which we have heretofore only guessed and many of which we have never fully understood. The science of electroencephalography, for example, despite its presence on the scene for a good many years, is still not completely mapped out. It is quite possible that we are overlooking a valuable scientific addition in depreciating some of the ancient Chinese beliefs of life energy or the parapsychologist's postulation of energy flow through the body.

The Chinese call their medicine *chi hua,* "the science of life," and this is what they mean when they say that acupuncture is a system of energy, and that energy, *chi,* is part of the sum and substance of the living organism, and that the phenomena of sickness and health can be explained in terms of disturbances of this energy. Skeptics may choose to call this idea simplistic. Perhaps—but it may also be too sophisticated. In ancient occidental times a man would stand on earth, watch the sun move from east to west, and claim that the earth is the center of the solar system and the sun revolves around it. Subsequent studies show how wrong he was. Future research will determine whether the ancient idea of *chi* is or

*We mention this in the question and answer section and are repeating it for emphasis.

is not antiquated, because it is quite obvious that someone's point of view is in error.

In conclusion, let me repeat my assertion: There is no "anatomy" of an acupuncture point. There are no acupuncture points. There are points which, on stimulation, can produce an acupuncture effect known not only in China but also in this country under a variety of names. This acupuncture effect can be initiated and transmitted in a variety of ways, but it is more specific, economical, and easily controlled when produced by needle-puncture along nervous pathways. It has a demonstrable physiologic effect on various parameters of the homeostatic organism. It can be shown to affect the progress of a disease. We shall hear a great deal more about this in the years to come from investigations being conducted here, in China, and elsewhere in the world.

(From an address at the New York University Medical Center teaching symposium "Acupuncture '73.")

Excerpt from the *Medical Tribune*, March 15, 1975:

Acupuncture Pain Relief Indicated to Be Independent of Site of Needle Insertion

WINNIPEG, MAN.—Preliminary results of a study of 91 acupuncture patients with chronic pain indicate that relief is not dependent on the site of needle insertion and that there is no more relief when the patients can look at the therapists than when they cannot.

Dr. Charles Godfrey, director of rehabilitation medicine, Wellesley Hospital, Toronto, reported these results to the annual meeting of the Royal College of Physicians and Surgeons of Canada.

A total of 82 percent of the patients experienced noticeable relief, 69 percent considerable relief, 61 percent considerable and lasting relief, and 30 percent had their pain reduced "very significantly" to only 10 percent of what it had been before, Dr. Godfrey said.

CHAPTER III

ELECTRICAL STIMULATION OF SKIN, PERIPHERAL NERVES, AND SPINAL DORSAL COLUMNS FOR CONTROL OF PAIN:

A 6½-YEAR EXPERIENCE

C. Norman Shealy, M.D.

Director, The Pain Rehabilitation Center, S.C.

Since our first dorsal column stimulator implant in April, 1967, we have seen over 1,600 chronic pain patients. Most of these have been tested with transcutaneous nerve stimulation; 21 have had implanted a variety of peripheral nerve stimulators, and 80 have had inserted dorsal column stimulators. We have also inserted 2 peripheral nerve stimulators and 10 dorsal column stimulators while visiting other neurosurgical centers; not all of these were screened by us and could not easily be followed by us. So, these 12 will not be included in subsequent statistics.

When a chronic pain patient is initially reviewed, he has usually been seen earlier by at least 4 other physicians, has had an average of 5 surgical procedures related to his pain, has had pain for 2 to 30 years and has had average medical costs of $50,000 to $75,000. In general, he has been overdiagnosed and overtreated, both with drugs and surgery.

Therefore, when we see a patient, we review his lengthy history and perform a general and neurologic exam. In only a few patients is it necessary to consider any elaborate special diagnostic aids. The physical problem has ordinarily been well defined.

Approximately 60% of such chronic pain patients have had one or multiple lumbar laminectomies with or without fusion. In general, in these patients, the diagnosis is obvious; many have complicating arachnoiditis; all have at least a modicum of epidural scar.

In our personal series, through the vagaries of referral patterns, cancer pain has represented about 2% of patients seen. About 2% are phantom limb pain syndrome, and an equal number have paraplegia. Post-surgical incisional pain, post-herpetic pain and a wide variety of other traumatic insults make up 1 or 2% of our pain population. Various forms of osteoarthritis make up about 10% of our pain patients. We discourage some referrals of arthritis patients, so this ratio is artificially low; otherwise we might well become an "arthritis clinic."

We have seen no value in most "diagnostic" nerve blocks; we neither recommend nor perform most destructive pain procedures. Thus, our primary approach is to accomplish symptomatic pain control in patients where the primary physical abnormality is not correctable. Obviously when we see "virgin" (i.e., unoperated) patients, greater attention is directed at ascertaining physical "causes."

Once the decision is made to treat the pain symptomatically, each patient is subjected to psychological evaluation through the MMPI (Minnesota Multiphasic Personality Inventory) and special pain questionnaire, and a personal survey by the physicians. Whenever an implanted stimulator is considered, psychiatric consultation is also obtained.

All patients are then treated with external transcutaneous electrical stimulation, applied to various parts of the body but especially concentrating upon the area of pain. The external stimulator currently used puts out a spike wave form similar to a nerve action potential. It has an 80-microsecond pulse width (at 50% amplitude), develops a peak current of 85 mamp (but develops less than 10 mamp effective heating value), and has variable frequency of 10 to 200 Hertz. Patients are initially subjected to TNS as much of the time as possible in 24 hours. Whenever simple application of the electrodes is not adequate, combinations of electrodes are tried and occasionally experimental paint-on electrodes are used.

With electrical stimulation, however applied, the patient feels a tingling, buzzing, vibrating sensation, spreading to various degrees peripheral to the electrode. Although partial pain relief may be reported when the tingling is not referred to the area of pain, *total* pain control has been seen only when the painful area has adequate sensation of stimulation. The sensation to the area of pain preferably should be adjusted to be stronger than that felt in non-painful parts.

In acute pain, such TNS is effective in accomplishing major pain control about 80% of the time. But in chronic pain only about 25% of patients find TNS adequate as the major therapy for their pain. About 50% more achieve partial relief. The pleasant exceptions are causalgia and post-herpetic pain, which experience excellent pain control about 60% of the time, with another 15% achieving partial relief.

	% of patients achieving pain relief		
	Poor	Fair (incomplete)	Good to Excellent
Acute (surgical wounds, fractures, sprains, etc.)	20	20	60
Parturition			
Back Pain	25		75
Perineal Pain	80	10	10
Chronic Pain			
Post herpetic	25	15	60
Phantom limb	40	35	25
Back Pain (Representing 60% of chronic patients)	25	50	25
Sciatic Pain (Representing 60% of chronic patients)	60	30	10
Neck Pain	50	25	25
Headaches	60	20	20
Arm & Hand Pain (including causalgia)	25	25	50
Diffuse Pain	80	10	10
Face Pain	50	25	25

Good to excellent pain control allows withdrawal of drugs and increasing physical activity.

Thus, acute pain, which represents the greatest volume of patients, also responds best to TNS. When we consider the nearly 3 billion aspirin tablets consumed each year the potential for an alternative therapy is obvious.

Although most chronic pain is not totally controlled by TNS, psychological factors and greater mobility complicate the clinical picture.

A decision about the effectiveness or failure of TNS is made within 2 weeks, during which time drugs are withdrawn and patients are subjected to an elaborate behavioral modification program, with great emphasis upon emotional attunement, and use of acupuncture and a variety of mechanical techniques to assist pain control. In the back patients, consideration is then given percutaneous electrocoagulative denervation of tender spinal facets.

Only after all these fail to accomplish acceptable pain control in patients considered to be reasonable stable emotionally should the possibility of implanted electronic stimulators be entertained.

When the pain is fairly focal, percutaneous electrical needle stimulation of appropriate nerves is tried. Simple hypo needles or spinal needles are used, placed near the nerve and attached to the TNS for stimulation for 30 to 60 minutes. When 90-100% pain relief is accomplished, the procedure is repeated at least two more times. Only then is implantation considered.

The following have been done:

	Total	Failures	Successes
Sciatic	16	7	9
Ulnar	1	0	1
Peroneal	2	1	1
Greater occipital	2	1	1

Thus, despite rigid screening, good control of pain in these patients has been accomplished only 57% of the time. Failure has been related to almost immediate lack of stimulation throughout the distribution of the nerve. Obviously, our screening electrode, crude though it is, is superior to the implanted electrode in delivering electrical current.

Finally, and when we and the patient are desperate, we entertain the possibility of an implanted DCS. During the first few years of this work we sometimes implanted DCS despite our opinion of a severely disturbed personality.

Surgeon's Opinion of Patient

1 Normal		2 Moderately Abnormal		3 Severely Abnormal	
Success	Failure	Success	Failure	Success	Failure
17	10	25	12	3	13

At this point we can only hope that our colleagues will heed this warning, since a success rate of 3 in 16 is totally unacceptable, and only the worst masochist would persist with such patients, for they are extremely difficult to manage. The MMPI yields similar results:

MMPI

Abnormal*		Normal**	
Success	Failure	Success	Failure
5	11	26	16

*Abnormal = 4 or more elevations of 70 or more
**Normal = 3 or less elevations of 70 or more

In addition to the clear-cut mandate to choose patients on the basis of personality, we have emphasized the requirement of a satisfactory test with electrical stimulation. Most of the time this is accomplished with TNS, which is found to provide partial pain relief and to be a tolerable sensation. The incomplete control usually reflects inability to accomplish electrical sensation (buzzing or tingling) in part of the area of pain, at least during activity.

When TNS leads to essentially no pain relief, but when the sensation is acceptable to the patient, percutaneous DCS is tried. This takes two forms:

In paraplegics (and rarely otherwise) we use *direct* cord stimulation, with a 0.012-inch electrode, electrically shielded except for a 2-mm. tip, passed through a 19-gauge spinal needle directly into the cord. Usually, we place the electrode in the thoracic cord, under X-ray guidance, 1 to 4 levels above the spinal cord lesion. This is done through mid-line posterior sagittal placement. When this is not feasible, we use the technique of Adams and Hosobuchi of a lateral C1-2 approach. With the lateral approach, stimulation continues for 20 to 30 minutes, but with paraplegics the thoracic electrode is left in position 1 to 2 hours.

We feel this test is minimally acceptable, as even an hour is too brief a time for patients to be certain such stimulation is accomplishing pain relief. About two-thirds of patients tested in this way choose to proceed to an implanted DCS.

More commonly we insert through a Touhy needle a "floating" flexible electrode which is placed either in the lumbar area and threaded up as cephalad as possible or behind the cord at C1-2 through a lateral approach. Stimulation of this electrode allows the test to be continued 24-48 hours, during which time the patient may walk around and provide a greater chance to be certain of effectiveness. Usually the tingling sensation can be well felt in only half the body and in one leg (or arm and leg). Only when the patient reports 90-100% pain relief in the area stimulated do we proceed to an implanted DCS. About 50% of the patients subjected to this percutaneous test elect to proceed. This low rate undoubtedly reflects the fact that most such patients have not achieved relief with TNS either. Implanted patients who have been screened in this way have an 85% success rate. So it is likely that we should recommend this test as the final hurdle in most patients. There have been no infections or neurologic complications with the percutaneous tests; but post-spinal headache is common.

In addition to personality and electrical stimulation, certain other factors have been found to have a major influence.

Conditions present prior to implant

Condition	Success	Failure
Cancer	4	2
Cordotomy	4	8
Cingulumotomy	0	4

Thus, it seems especially essential that percutaneous DCS be done in patients who have had previous cordotomy. Such patients should be chosen for implanted DCS only when personality is quite stable and when percutaneous DCS gives total pain relief. Even then great attention must be paid to the placement of the DCS electrode which should, with unilateral cordotomy patients, be placed 2 to 3 mm. *toward* the *side of pain*. Otherwise, excess stimulation will be *felt* on the side of the cordotomy lesion or the non-painful side!

Our results in patients with a previous cingulumotomy force us to conclude that such patients should not be implanted. As already indicated, we believe cordotomy and cingulumotomy should not be done for chronic benign pain.

There is slight difference in results in males and females.

Sex of patient as related to success or failure

	Male	Female
Success	24	21
Failure	21	14
	45	35 = 80

Electrode placement is crucial. With electrodes used to date subdural, extra-arachnoid placement has been most satisfactory. Endodural placement, within layers of the dura, has led to inadequate stimulation and to excess stimulation in the area nearest the electrode. Our personal experience has not included endodural placement of bipolar electrodes, reported by Dr. Charles Burton to be quite satisfactory in this location. Although the number is small, epidural electrode placement has been as satisfactory as subdural and should be investigated further.

Electrode placement

Placement	Success	Failure
Epidural	4	2
Endodural	5	8
Subdural	54	34
	63	44 = 107

The *type* of electrode is even more crucial.

Type of electrode implanted

Electrode	Success	Failure
Avery bipolar	0	1
Tripolar	23	12
Bipolar tinsel	13	12
Monopolar tinsel	25	19
Monopolar plate	2	0
	63	44 = 107

Combinations of electrode type and placement

Placement	Electrode	Success	Failure
Epidural	Tripolar	2	0
	Bipolar tinsel	1	1
	Monopolar tinsel	1	1
Endodural	Tripolar	1	0
	Bipolar tinsel	1	0
	Monopolar tinsel	3	8
Subdural	Tripolar	19	12
	Avery bipolar	0	1
	Bipolar tinsel	11	11
	Monopolar tinsel	22	10
	Monopolar plate	2	0
		63	44 = 107

Although the numbers are not of statistical significance, the implications are important and in practice even the "successful" patients with tinsel wire electrodes have not fared as well as those with solid platinum plates. Note that we have placed 107 electrodes in 80 patients to allow comparison of two different electrodes.

Our overall success rate in only 56% of patients reflects a variety of problems.

Reasons for failure

Reason	Frequency of Occurrence
Personality	19
Paraplegia (from DCS)	2
Inadequate stimulation and type electrode	4
Neurologic deficit (pre-existing paraplegia)	2
Electrode placement	1
Uncertain	3
Personality (cingulumotomy)	4
	35

Note: six more patients were added to the problem personality category (whereas we had considered 16 patients in this category originally, only 3 achieved pain relief with DCS); six patients who had appeared to be fair candidates became so hysterical, hostile, and obstreperous that we had to assume that our assessment was wrong (in every such instance, the MMPI had supplied the clue so if we had combined a "fair" opinion with a "poor" MMPI, the patient would not have been done).

Through a complicated system of correlations we find that only 17 of the 45 successful patients have returned to normal work without drugs. The other 28 had all been off work more than two years and most had pre-existing complicating physical or neurotic deficits. It seems unreasonable to expect most paraplegics, amputees, and partially paralyzed patients to return to "normal" activity. Even in patients admitting marked pain improvement, drug reduction has not been as great as desirable. To a large extent these are tranquilizers and not analgetics.

The pain etiologies in our DCS group are virtually the same as in the general chronic pain patients.

Pain Etiology	Success	Failure
Failures of disc surgery	31	17
Cancer	5	2
Arachnoiditis	3	2
Paraplegia	3	5
Phantom limb	1	4
Thalamic pain syndrome	1	0
Tabes dorsalis	0	1
Crush injury of leg	0	1
Cauda equina trauma	1	1
Post surgical	0	1
Unknown pain cause	0	1
	45	35

Complications

A tremendous variety of complications has been seen in the DCS patients.

Type of complication	Frequency of occurrence
CSF leak	16
Electrode removed	5
Prolonged pain associated with operative wounds	10
Poor localization, inadequate stimulation	12
Hematoma, incisional (minor)	5
Uncomfortable paresthesia	7
Mechanical problems, requiring re-operation, re-positioning, or repair of wire	15
Partial paraplegia	3
Infection	1
Seroma	3

Total number of patients with complications = 48
Total number of complications = 77

Fortunately, most of the problems have not been serious, but four patients (5%) have had life-threatening or life-incapacitating threats (infections or paraplegias). Of these, all four have partially or totally recovered. All three of the paraparetic problems occurred with a tripolar electrode measuring about 78 microns thickness and having a rather rigid right angle lead wire take-off. The thickness has been reduced to 60 microns in these leads and the electrode wire has been returned to our original 45-degree angle with a thinner wire. Hopefully, this will obviate such complications. Epidural electrode placement must also be further evaluated, as it would offer the greatest mechanical safety.

Nevertheless, these risks and potential risks offer a potent argument against indiscriminate use of this procedure, which was introduced in an attempt to offer a safe, non-destructive technique for pain relief. All the other complications are relatively minor technical, mechanical problems which can be avoided with care, experience and with potential improvements in the equipment. Late electrical problems have been uncommon but undoubtedly will increase with more time. No late neurologic problems have been seen.

Whenever adequate stimulation is not referred to the area of pain, variations in pulse width and in frequency are tried. In some patients special transmitters supplying either a ramp or a cycling pattern of stimulation have been valuable assistants and have converted a failure to a reasonable success. In a small number of patients both the pulse rate and/or the pulse width have crucial restricted requirements for successful pain relief. Such trouble-shooting is time-consuming but essential in managing these patients.

Summary

Screening of chronic pain patients with TNS is quite worthwhile as it leads to useful control of pain in 25% of patients and to partial control in another 50%. In the 75% who do not obtain complete or nearly complete control with TNS, further treatment and evaluation with MMPI, acupuncture, personal interviews, behavioral modification and mechanical stimulations, serious consideration is given to either an implanted peripheral nerve stimulator or, in about 1% of patients, a DCS. Percutaneous needle stimulation of peripheral nerve or percutaneous flexible electrode for DCS offers the final selection process. Only 5% of 200 chronic pain patients have been selected for such implants. Fifty-seven percent of the 21 peripheral nerve implants have achieved adequate pain control. Fifty-six percent of the DCS patients have satisfactory (marked to excellent) pain control. Patients who have had cingulumotomy and those with recognized severe personality problems should be excluded. If we had exercised these criteria, our DCS success rate would have been 70%. Modification in electrode and its positioning probably would have raised the success rate above 80%. Many minor complications are correctable by technical care and exercise. The 5% rate of serious, potentially devastating complications can, hopefully, be reduced by improvements in electrode design; but the potential risk remains to remind us that any open surgical procedure for control of benign pain must be undertaken only as a last resort. No patient has died and none in our series has yet been rendered permanently paraplegic; but one patient remains paraparetic six months after surgery. DCS has passed the five-year mark but is in the developmental stage with a number of technical problems still to be improved. And our original desire of a percutaneously implanted electrode has yet to be designed.

CHAPTER IV

TWENTY-SEVEN ACUPUNCTURE POINTS: THEIR ELECTRICAL RESISTANCE

Norman L. Wulfsohn; James H. K. Yoo; Jerry Gelineau

Departments of Anesthesiology and Bioengineering. The University of Texas Health Science Center, San Antonio, Texas.

Acupuncture, known for over 5,000 years in the Orient, is derived from the words *acus* (needle) and *punctura* (puncture). Very fine needles are inserted into the skin at specific points on the body. Only in recent years have the Chinese found that these points can be located electrically. When a pencil probe is passed over these areas a reduced electrical resistance is noted compared to the surrounding skin (Mann). However, the electrical resistance of these points has not been systematically measured and recorded. The purpose of this study was to determine this parameter at various sites.

Method

To measure the electrical resistance of the selected acupuncture points an 1/8-inch probe was used. It had a gold plated blunt point and small weights were applied to the probe to give it good skin contact. The probe weighed 40.0 gm for measurement in the males, and 35.0 gm for measurement in the females. When measuring the acupuncture point on the ear, less weight was used (17.0 gm) to avoid damage to the softer and more tender skin.

Measurements were made in eight healthy volunteers, four female, and four male. Excluded were persons on any type of medication or who were pregnant. Electrical resistance was measured in kilo-ohms (KΩ) by passing a 50 μ amp current through the skin. A graphic record was made using a Grass Polygraph, Model 7. The positive electrode was connected to the thumb, big toe, or neck, for measurement on the arm, leg, or ear, respectively. Twenty-seven acupuncture sites were measured, chosen from meridianal points on the upper limb, lower limb or ear. At least two points were chosen from each meridian. (Fig. 1)

The probe was lightly brushed over the skin in approximately the anatomical location of each acupuncture point until an area of low resistance was found. This resistance was then measured. The surrounding skin area was also measured for comparison, starting about ¼ of an inch lateral to the acupuncture point, trying to avoid the direct line of the meridianal path. Sometimes the lower electrical resistance was not circumscribed to a point but rather an area of about ½ inch or, in some instances, one inch. In these cases the skin resistance for control purposes was noted outside these acupuncture areas.

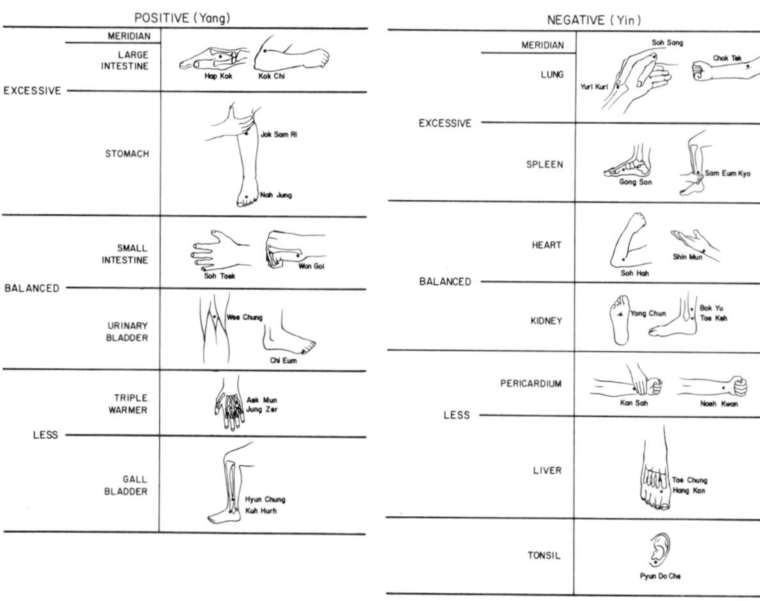

Fig. 1. The Anatomical Locations of the 27 Acupuncture Points; Modified from the Shanghai Acupuncture Research Institute.

In some instances when the probe was applied to the acupuncture point the response was rapid, only a few seconds being required for the resistance to fall to its lowest level. In others it took longer. This rate of response was related to the fatness of the individual, as determined from Weisberg's formula:

% fat = 90-2 (height-girth) of body weight (height = inches, girth = inches, measured at the umbilical level).

Results

The mean electrical resistance of the 27 acupuncture points in eight persons (total of 216 points) was 794 ± 179 KΩ and of the control areas 1407 ± 306 KΩ, a 56% difference and statistically significant, $p < 0.001$. This difference between acupuncture points and control areas, in males and females, and in different parts of the body is shown in Table I and Figures 2 and 3.

In men and women there is a difference between the same acupuncture points ($p = 0.005$) but not in the control points ($p = 0.4$). Also there is a difference between the acupuncture points in the upper limb and the lower limb ($p = 0.005$) but not between the hand and arm, nor the foot and leg. Points on the same meridian varied one from another in their electrical resistance in the same individual. Some could be considered "strong" points (low resistance) and others "weak" points (higher resistance). (Table II.)

In some cases the rate of descent of the recording to its lowest level was rapid, in others slower. These persons could thus be designated as "slow responders" or "fast responders." The fast responders are fatter, having a higher percentage of fat in their body weight. (See Fig. 4.) A linear regression curve, obtained by the least square method, is given in the figure

$$(y \simeq -0.86x + 30.12; \quad \gamma = 0.94).$$

Table I. Summarized Data of the Skin Resistance of the 27 Acupuncture Points and the Controlled Sites

	Acupuncture*	Controlled*	Difference*	% Difference	Significance Level
μ average	795	1407	612	56	<0.001
μ men	831	1419	588	52	<0.001
μ women	759	1396	637	59	<0.001
	μ men*	**μ women***	**Difference***		
Acup.	831	759	-72	-6	0.005
Cont.	1419	1396	-23	-2	0.4
Average	1125	1078	-47	-4	0.1
	μ upper limb*	**μ lower limb***	**Difference***		
Acup.	780	849	69	8	0.005
Cont.	1316	1553	237	17	0.001
Average	1048	1201	153	12	0.001
	μ hand*	**μ arm***	**Difference***		
Acup.	807	753	-54	-6	0.1
Cont.	1270	1356	86	7	0.5
Average	1038	1054	16	2	0.7
	μ foot*	**μ leg***	**Difference***		
Acup.	890	814	-76	-9	0.05
Cont.	1528	1578	50	3	0.2
Average	1209	1196	-13	1	0.8

*All values are in KΩ units.

Table II. Variations of the Skin Resistances of the 27 Acupuncture Points and the Controlled Sites

Meridians		Lung			Spleen		Heart		Kidney			Pericard-ium		Liver		Large Intestine		Stomach		Small Intestine		Urinary Bladder		Triple Warmer		Gall Bladder		Tonsil
Names**		SS	YK	CT	GS	SEK	SH	SM	YC	TK	BY	KS	NK	HKN	TC	HKK	KC	JSR	NJ	ST	WG	NC	CE	AM	JZ	HZ	KH	PDC
Locations***		H	A	A	F	L	A	A	F	L	L	A	A	F	F	H	A	L	F	H	H	L	F	H	H	L	L	E
Acupuncture Points	$\overline{X}_8$	491	794	675	925	969	569	725	1000	788	794	915	915	788	1000	788	675	931	713	744	1031	825	913	1100	688	550	838	313
	$\overline{X}_{men}$	495	713	750	863	1325	613	700	1050	825	788	1113	930	700	1013	763	750	1088	613	500	963	1125	775	1450	638	663	838	388
	$\overline{X}_{women}$	488	875	600	988	613	525	750	950	750	800	718	900	875	988	813	600	775	813	988	1100	525	1050	750	738	438	838	238
Controlled Points	$\overline{X}_8$	906	1231	1219	1469	1531	1075	1563	1588	1850	1613	1363	1669	1025	1650	1475	1369	1956	1450	1250	1384	1600	1388	1388	1219	1113	1381	488
	$\overline{X}_{men}$	787	1263	1375	1663	1975	1313	1450	1425	1950	1625	1500	1363	1400	1625	1330	1250	2000	1325	800	1243	1900	1425	1150	1263	1625	1325	675
	$\overline{X}_{women}$	1025	1230	1063	1275	1088	838	1675	1750	1750	1600	1225	1975	1850	1675	1600	1488	1913	1575	1700	1525	1300	1350	1625	1175	600	1438	300

*All values are in KΩ units

**Refer to Fig. 1 for names of acupuncture points.

***H:Hand; A:Arm; F:Foot; L:Leg

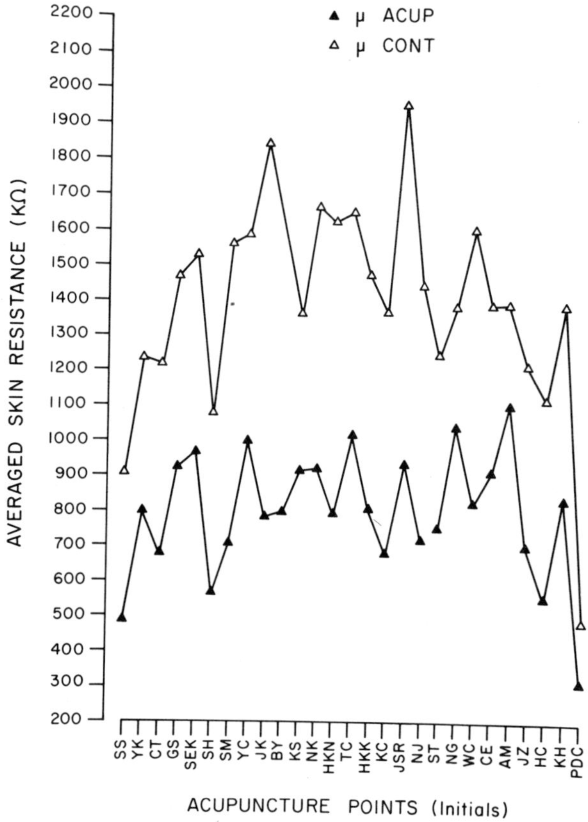

Fig. 2. Skin Resistance at Acupuncture Points and Controlled Sites
Acup = Acupuncture Points; Cont = Control Points

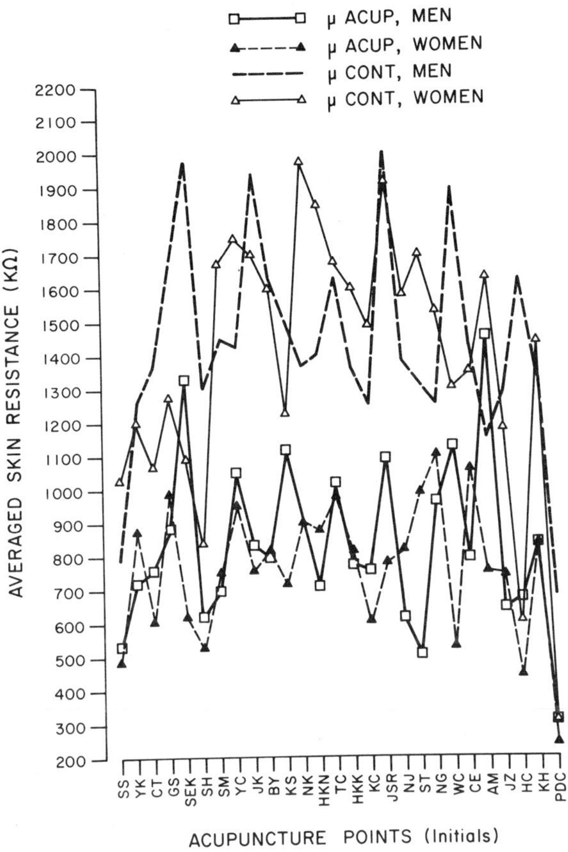

Fig. 3. Skin Resistance for Men and Women
Acup = Acupuncture Points; Cont = Control Points

Discussion

There are about one thousand acupuncture points described, mostly reflecting the activity of the visceral organs. These points are distributed in twelve bilateral meridians or lines running from chest to distal parts of arm, leg, or head. The meridians are designated as *Yin* or *Yang*, having qualities of positivity or negativity, or perhaps sympathetonia or parasympathetonia. The *Yin* meridians represent "solid organs" (lung, heart, sex organs, spleen, liver, kidney) and the *Yang* meridians the "hollow organs" (large intestine, small intestine, stomach, gall bladder, urinary bladder, etc.). The meridians run in three meridianal cycles, starting in the anterior chest wall, and so on. Mann suggests the meridians follow the embryonic patterns of the development of the anterior and posterior surfaces of the body and limbs.

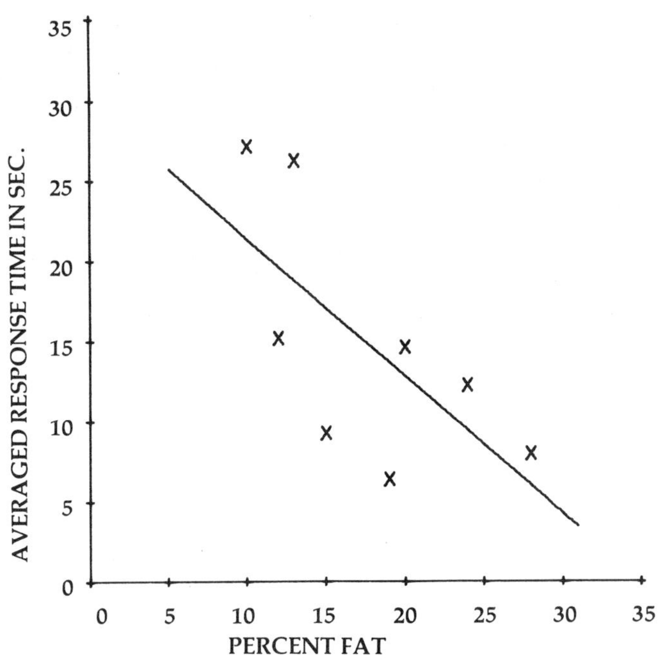

Fig. 4. Averaged Response Time vs. Percent Fat

Acupuncture points are generally located at specific anatomical points and require many years of experience to locate correctly. In disease states the acupuncturist finds these points by their tenderness to pressure, sometimes by whitish or purplish streaks along the meridian, or by some aedema, or by the development of a nodule at the site. With very light brushing of the fingers over the skin the experienced acupuncturist can soon locate the area.

However, these points can also be located electrically, as has been shown recently by the Chinese. In the present study, after finding the point by the change in electrical resistance compared to the surrounding skin, the resistance was measured. The resistance of 216 acupuncture points was in most cases lower than the surrounding skin areas. It was lower in women than in men and lower in the upper limb than the lower limb.

Others have also found electrical changes relating to acupuncture points. Using an alternating current the measured resistance at acupuncture points was found to be diminished (Mann). The audio-frequency conductivity and the electrical potential of the skin have been found to be greater at these sites than at the surrounding tissues (Mann).

It appears that acupuncture points are in some way joined together in a line, along the meridian. Stimulation of an acupuncture point affects the electrical activity of other acupuncture points on the same meridian (Mann). However, if the anatomical meridian is cut this increase of electrical activity is not present. Stimulation of an acupuncture point related to the large intestine will cause an increase of peristalsis in rabbits in about one minute. If the anatomical meridian is cut this does not happen (Mann). In reverse, electrical stimulation of the stomach caused an alteration in the electrical resistance of certain acupuncture points (Mann). And conversely, stimulation of certain points in the ear caused a change of electrical resistance over the abdomen (Dimond, 1971). This could be due to factors that influence the electrical resistance of the skin such as subcutaneous fat, texture of skin or blood flow to the skin. No correlation was found to percentage fat in this study, although there is a correlation of electrical resistance with amount of subcutaneous fat (Geddes). The ear, which has a softer and thinner skin, had a lower resistance than the limbs. However, one cannot say why in the same individual acupuncture points vary in electrical resistance on the same meridian, although it is known that there are so-called strong and weak acupuncture points.

Sweat gland activity also affects the electrical resistance of the skin. In the present study the volunteers were measured in a cool, airconditioned room and were in a relaxed and calm mood. Changes in mental status can affect the electrical activity of the skin, presumably partly by their effect on sweat glands. The agitated depressive has a higher level of electrical resistance of the skin than normal, whereas the retarded depressive has a low lever (Lader and Wing; Noble and Lader). Deep breathing, auditory stimuli and superficial nerve stimulation can also cause a transitory increase in galvanic skin resistance (Filmer, 1971; Lader and Wing).

Electrical conductance of skin is also an indicator of stress, it being increased in stress, whether the stress is anticipated or not (Opton).

Summary

The electrical resistance of the skin at 27 acupuncture points in 8 volunteers was measured. Of the total of 216 points examined the average resistance was 794 $\pm$ 179 KΩ and of the skin surrounding the acupuncture points 1407 $\pm$ 306 KΩ, a 56% difference. The resistance of acupuncture points is lower in women than men, lower in the upper limb than the lower limb. In some volunteers the minimum level of resistance was reached rapidly, in others slowly, and thus they were designated as fast or slow responders. The fast responders are fatter than the slow responders.

REFERENCES

1. Dimond, E.G. Modern Education and Care in People's Republic of China. J. Amer. Med. Assoc. 218: 1558-1563, 1971.
2. Geddes, L.A. *Electrodes and The Measurement of Biolective Events.* John Wiley and Sons, New York, 1972.
3. Fuhrer, M.J. Skin conductance responses mediated by the transected human spinal cord. J. Appl. Physiol. 30: 663-9, 1971.
4. Lader, M. H. and Wing, L. Physiological measures in agitated and retarded depressed patients. J. Psychiatr. Res. 7: 89-100, 1969.
5. Mann, F. *Acupuncture, The Ancient Chinese Art of Healing.* Random House, New York, 1972.
6. Noble, P. and Lader, M. The symptomatic correlates of the skin conductance changes in depression. J. Psychiatr. Res. 9: 61-69, 1971.
7. Opton, E. Psychological stress and coping processes in the practice of dentistry. Int. Dental. J. 19: 415-429, 1969.
8. Weisberg, H. F. *Water, Electrolyte and Acid-Base Balance.* 3rd Ed. Baltimore, The Williams and Wilkins Co., 1972.
9. Shanghai Acupuncture Research Institute. *Simple, Concise Acupuncture Methods of Treatment.* The Academy Press Co., Hong Kong, 1969.

CHAPTER V

ACUPUNCTURE AND CHINESE PHILOSOPHY

David Saltoun, M.B.Ch.B., B.O.A., D.A.

Consulting Anesthesiologist

It is easy to disparage acupuncture as propaganda, hypnosis, or twaddle, but it is not easy to forget that it is one of the principal ingredients of Chinese medicine, to which the inhabitants of this vast country turn as naturally as we do to aspirin.

China, with a population of 800 million people, has now finally opened her doors to the West. In March and April of 1972, on a Medical Study Visit, Chinese medicine, surgery, obstetrics, and anesthetics practiced in the major teaching hospitals in Peking, Canton, Nanking, Shanghai, and Wuhsi were all observed. The accelerated health program following the liberation in 1949 and the great proletarian Cultural Revolution of 1966 generated medical programs and methods which may seem strange to the Western-oriented physician, but for China and the Chinese, it definitely works. Their policy has been to blend traditional Chinese medicine and conventional Western therapy. Together with a massive public health program, it has produced spectacular results in the cities as well as the urban areas.

It is nothing short of a monumental achievement, especially if one looks at the communities in the country districts and sees how their health service is organized. Tracing this up through varying degrees of sophistication in the universities and medical schools and to the training of the students, we understand a great many additional facets concerning the circumscribed procedures of acupuncture and acupuncture anesthesia.

In farming regions, communes have been built, each with about seventy-five to one hundred thousand peasants. The Chinese favor and frequently utilize "peasants" in speech and in writing. Communes are primarily engaged in growing food for themselves and for sale to the urban areas. Each commune has its own hospital with between 50 and 100 beds and a staff of physicians and surgeons trained in the Western manner. Nurses and traditional doctors are drawn from the community. These hospitals can handle routine minor illnesses as well as emergency surgical procedures. Their capability extends to procedures such as gastrointestinal perforation, appendectomy, and caesarean section. Each is equipped with an operating theater which primarily uses acupuncture anesthesia for operative procedures. The pharmacies are equipped with ion exchange resin columns, so that they can produce their own fluids for intravenous infusion. The pharmacies also have methods of producing ampules to contain their own locally produced vitamin extracts and anti-inflammatory agents for intravenous injection. Tablet-making machines are also installed so that tablet medication can be produced from the local traditional herbal remedies. Patients with complicated and difficult conditions are transferred to the more sophisticated larger district hospitals and, if need be, to the hospitals associated with the medical schools. There are now approximately one million "barefoot doctors" in China. The day-to-day care of the peasants is performed by these barefoot doctors, who essentially are peasant workers with only a simple three-week training in medical diagnosis and treatment, usually traditional, who act both as a filter for disease beyond their capability of treating or as the therapist for simple conditions of influenza, chronic bronchitis, and minor ailments. The barefoot doctor gets a three-week refresher course at the local hospital every year. The barefoot doctor or his counterpart, the worker-doctor in the factory communes, forms the backbone of the basic minor health care and education of the peasant. (Each commune has a woman barefoot doctor who is responsible for the contraceptive advice to the women of the community. Contraception is highly advanced with Chinese-made contraceptive pills as well as intrauterine contraceptive devices.) It should be noted that being a barefoot doctor is not the sole occupation of that person, as he still has to be a food-producing member of his commune production brigade.

In China today, great emphasis has been placed on traditional medicine. The emphasis is evident by the names of the three major hospital departments: 1. Department of Traditional Medicine; 2. Department of Western Medicine; and 3. Department of Combined Western and Traditional Medicine.

Even more important is that the patient has freedom of choice as to which department he attends. Despite the figures of twenty-five hundred to three thousand patients per day, patients moved freely between departments even when the diagnosis was made by the respective doctors.

1. *Department of Traditional Medicine:* Staffed by traditional medical doctors who have graduated from a traditional medical college. Period of training: three years. He learns the art of pulse diagnosis and examining the tongue, but he also takes a history. Therapy takes the form of traditional herbal remedies. The presumption is to correct the state of imbalance which has arisen and hence produced the symptoms. Some of this traditional treatment has been modernized. Injections and tablets made from the extracts of herbs are often given. Chronic bronchitis, peptic ulceration, menorrhagia, and heart conditions are common conditions given traditional medicine as the major form of therapy. Acupuncture is the other principal ingredient of traditional treatment.

Many Western-trained Chinese doctors have been treated with acupuncture needles for relief of headaches, possibly of tension origin. Interestingly enough, while these doctors know the points of insertion of these needles, *they do not treat themselves* but have other people, for example their wives or relatives, insert the needles for them. The insertion of needles is practiced by lay people almost the same way that the average person in a Western country would take an aspirin tablet. In the Children's Palace in Shanghai, young children practice inserting needles into one another's arms, legs , and faces to become proficient both as a user and as a recipient. In the Traditional Department of the hospital, therefore, acupuncture therapy was constantly utilized. Two typical cases are as follows: 1) Treatment of peptic ulceration: Needles were placed into the lower one-third of the leg and into the anterior wall of the abdomen, and a galvanic current was passed. The site of emplacement of the needles in this instance was located by the use of an electronic stimulator to find the most sensitive area. 2) The after-effects of poliomyelitis were treated by inserting ¼-inch pieces of catgut into the wasted muscles twice a week for ten weeks through a long hollow French's needle. A desirable effect was obviously attained.

2. *Department of Western Medicine:* The technical expertise of the Chinese surgeon, as would be expected, was superb. Such operations as thyroidectomy, gastrectomy, pneumonectomy, caesarean section, and intestinal resection, which were performed

with the patient under acupuncture anesthesia, were observed. One department in Shanghai and another in Nanking showed several fully-healed patients and some healing examples of limb reattachment. The limbs, as shown, were not merely embellishments but performed as a useful, functioning part with excellent movement, grip, and sensation. It was sad to see that while an excellent restorative operation could be performed, the prophylactic safety conditions in the factories visited were truly noticeable by their absence. Several burned patients were seen in whom extensive grafting had taken place, but unfortunate contractures of fingers and wrists were seen where no concurrent physiotherapy was being performed. Delivery in the labor rooms was by the suction method. Caesarean section was by lower segment approach.

3. *Department of Combined Western and Traditional Medicine:* This type of department will probably be the future typical Chinese medical approach. Traditional Chinese medicine and methodology are being taught to the present day medical student. *One must be wary of interpretation of reports from these departments claimed by lay visitors, since sensational therapy could be mistaken by those who are unaware of the natural pathology of many conditions.*

Many patients with appendicitis are treated by traditional therapy, but the Western-trained surgeon himself monitors these patients before traditional therapy is commenced and, if indicated, performs appendectomy. Similarly, ectopic pregnancy is treated by conservative means even after posterior colpotomy with a needle to establish the diagnosis. Both gallstones and renal calculi are treated by traditional means. Patients with stones were presented to us, along with the roentgenograms, and stones which had been passed or dissolved using traditional medicine. Fractures of the femur were treated by the insertion of a Steinmann pin through the tibial tubercle, but a Thomas splint was not applied. Instead, about ten pieces of wood, 10 by 1 by 1, were placed longitudinally around the site of fracture and held by a circumferential bandage which was adjusted daily. The patient was allowed to start bending his knee and to perform on his monkey frame as soon as it was possible to do so without causing pain. In these patients, both roentgenograms and patients demonstrated extremely good results with regard to muscle and joint function as well as in final position and callous formation.

Acupuncture Anesthesia

The surgical film released from China—and the recent appearance of reports in both the lay and medical United States press—of operations performed with patients under acupuncture anesthesia has aroused considerable interest and curiosity among the medical profession. The evolution of the technique as explained by the Chinese is that acupuncture therapy was used for the relief of pain and, hence, on this basis, if this therapy could alleviate pain could it not, therefore, be used to prevent pain during an operative procedure? Experiments were conducted to find new points in the body at which, if a needle were inserted, anesthesia could be produced. The points found were not necessarily the same as the classical points described under acupuncture therapy. Many of these points correspond to the course of the superficial sensory nerves. Acupuncture anesthesia consists of inserting a needle through the skin at a predetermined point in the body and applying a stimulus to the needle either by rotating it by hand or by passing a small specialized voltage current to produce a galvanic stimulation using the electrical box. After insertion, the stimulation is applied for 20 minutes prior to the commencement of the operation and is continued for the duration of the procedure. However, on many occasions, the acupuncturist would desist stimulating for many minutes while she carried out some other task, with no detriment in the anesthesia. Acupuncture anesthesia was started slowly in 1958, and began to gain increasing popularity from 1968. Apparently 80 percent of the Chinese population react to this form of anesthesia, while it fails in 20 percent. It should also be noted that not every operative procedure is capable of being performed under acupuncture anesthesia. For example, vaginal hysterectomy or a nailing procedure cannot be done. These procedures are usually done with the patient under spinal anesthesia, since general anesthesia equipment is somewhat sparsely distributed throughout China. In 14 hospitals visited we saw only two machines. Acupuncture anesthesia is probably a misnomer and should be called acupuncture analgesia. The patient does not fall asleep, and loses the sensation of pain only at the operative site while retaining the sensations of touch and the response to hot and cold at the site and elsewhere.

Chinese needles cost less than one cent each, and in many operations, especially thoracotomy, only one needle was observed to be used in the upper part of the arm. This could certainly compensate for the marked paucity of Western-type anesthetic machines and effect a huge savings in the supply of anesthetic gases necessary for this operation.

Most of the anesthesiologists seen using this method were not Western or traditional doctors but young girls who had been given a three-month course in the application of the needles. There were some Western-trained doctors applying the methods, and in the university hospitals most of the acupuncture anesthesiologists were under the supervision of a Western-trained doctor. Certainly, the Western-trained doctor kept an extremely wary eye not only on the acupuncturist but also on the patient while the operation was proceeding.

During the operative procedure, the patient remains conscious and in communication with the surgeon. This was useful in thyroidectomies where structures thought to be the recurrent laryngeal nerve were tested by clamping and getting the patient to speak before cutting the tissue. Similarly, reinflation of the lung after lobectomy was attained by the patient breathing on instruction from the acupuncturist in the manner in which he had been taught in the few days prior to the operation. During the pulmonary operations, which were lengthy, the patient usually ate pieces of apple or orange while talking to the operating room staff.

It was suggested that postoperative complications were lessened by acupuncture anesthesia. The postoperative complication rate was lower, and wounds healed more readily. I was impressed after an ovarian cystectomy in which the patient leaped from the trolley into her bed and preened herself for one minute prior to giving audience to her husband and young child, who were waiting for her outside the ward for her return from the operating room.

Disadvantages of Acupuncture Anesthesia

A thorough laparotomy cannot be conducted using this method of analgesia. In a gastrectomy, the surgeon is limited to the upper part of the abdomen and cannot feel down into the pelvis or examine the kidneys, as this would cause pain. The preoperative diagnosis, therefore, has to be 100 percent correct, as the surgeon cannot change his mind and perform a more radical procedure.

Because of the limited area of analgesia, the operations are of necessity conducted slowly. There is no undue pulling on the mesentery in abdominal operations, and the rib-spreader used during thoracotomy was opened slowly. If the pleura or peritoneum was stretched, the patient would grimace, sweat, and show some signs of shock, although in general the blood pressure and pulse rate would stay relatively static during the operation.

Acupuncture anesthesia tended to work better in nonemergency situations in which the patient had a few days' indoctrination prior to operation. Emergency operations were usually done under conventional spinal techniques.

The major question which arises is, Does acupuncture anesthesia work and, if so, how? It is extremely difficult to believe that the insertion of a needle and the stimulation of it will allow an extensive operation to take place without some adjunct therapy. Indeed, in many of the patients seen, adjunct therapy was given in the form of preoperative barbiturate medication, together with the intravenous administration of pethidine (meperidine) and Phenergan (promethazine hydrochloride) during the operation. There was also the application of surface-active local anesthetics to the rectus sheath and peritoneum, while in gastrectomy, injections of 1 percent procaine were made into the celiac plexus to aid the procedure. In the postoperative care of the patient, pethidine as well as an acupuncture needle was used to alleviate pain. The real question to be answered, therefore, is, which therapy, the acupuncture needle or the concomitant Western medication, is the adjunct? The care and patience with which the Chinese surgeon performs his operations, and the implicit faith of the patient, enable the dosages of barbiturate, pethidine, and local anesthetic to be lower than would be used normally in an excitable person. In neurosurgical operations, the scalp was well injected with 50 milliliters of local anesthetic before the incision was made, while the acupuncture needle was being stimulated in the patient's nasion.

In conclusion, it would seem that whether a patient gets well from traditional or Western medical methods is unimportant to the patient but becomes of great importance to the Western medical profession if there is some extra help we can give patients by adopting some of the Chinese methods. Acupuncture therapy has lasted more than 2,000 years. Acupuncture anesthesia is now in its infancy. The future will not see the exodus of the anesthetic machine, but rather the addition of a new and exciting modality to the physician's armamentarium.

My gratitude to Dr. Ian Copperauld for his cooperation in the preparation of this chapter.

D.S.

The Acupuncture Panorama

Why is a book on American acupuncture featuring the comments of a British anesthesiologist so prominently?

For one, Dr. Saltoun is probably the first anesthesiologist from the Western world to visit China and give us a close-hand impression. Second, the comments on analgesia that could be extracted from Dr. Dimond's article in the AMA *Journal*, while valuable, cannot carry the same authority as a report formulated by a specialist in the pain area. Third, Dr. Saltoun's opinion is untinged by favoritism or partiality to American pharmaceutical journalism.

It is with respect to this intimate knowledge of the system and of the present status of Chinese medicine, then, that we offer our classification of what I call the "acupuncture panorama."

As I have previously stated, there really are no acupunctural points; acupuncture is really not a circumscribed entity but is rather a catch-bag of effects—the acupuncture panorama. Not less than 15 techniques can be classified as productive of the acupunctural effect, and only half of these are Oriental. I hope that this statement will not throw the reader's thinking into disarray, but rather that it will open a new vista on this fascinating modality.

Chinese acupuncture is rarely, if ever, used alone; it is usually only one part of the treatment administered by a Chinese physician. The other parts can include diet, massage, herbs, exercise, deep breathing, and meditation. It is probably because of these concomitants that acupuncture works better in the Orient, and not because patients are ethnically motivated.

1. Antique or Ancient Chinese Acupuncture (2500-5000 years old)

Here acupuncture and its concomitants are part of tribal lore. The shaman, or tribal leader, who may have noticed the effect of flint arrows in reducing pains, is the doctor as well as the repository of these traditional ideas.

2. Classical Chinese Acupuncture

This amorphous material from many tribes and areas is codified into the Nei Ching by the Yellow Emperor and made the official medicine of the country.

3. Medieval Acupuncture

Acupuncture appears in France and Germany first and then takes hold in the rest of Europe in the seventh, eighth, and ninth centuries, disappearing shortly afterwards.

4. Modern Acupuncture

Acupuncture is widely practiced in all parts of the Orient, and diplomats from Western countries are exposed to it. In the period 1900-1920 it falls into disfavor, however, for two reasons: First, it has become very cultish and competitive—among its practitioners, one finds physicians with secret formulae and secret points; second, Western medical ideas are considered much more fashionable. Acupuncture declines steadily in the Orient, despite its reintroduction into France by Soulie de Morant, a diplomat, in 1930. Soon only "backward" (not barefoot) doctors are practicing it.

5. Neomodern or Revolutionary Acupuncture (about 1949)

Acupuncture is reinstated as an official state medical modality in China. It is again taught in the schools, and teams of regulation M.D.'s and "barefoot" acupuncturists, working together, are entrusted with the care of 800 million Chinese citizens.

6. Acupuncture Analgesia (about 1958)

A synaptic jump occurred in the brain of a Chinese physician, Li Chien, who postulated that if acupuncture can stop a toothache after the pain starts, perhaps it can prevent pain from starting if applied prophylactically before dental treatment. "Twirling" is thus introduced, and a new era of acupuncture begins, the era of electrification.

7. The Present Period of Acupuncture

The attachment of an electrical stimulator (#626) to the acupuncture needle heralds the beginning of a new era of experimentation and success in surgery. Acute attention must be paid to this period, in that contemporary acupuncture is completely different from ancient Chinese acupuncture; it is less than two decades old and is said by some to have derived from Japanese Ryodoraku, an electrical system devised by Dr. Nakatani eight years earlier (1950).

8. Moxibustion

An offshoot of acupuncture, moxibustion was developed in the Classical period and was used promiscuously in many forms—both with and without needles. It found favor in Japan as well, and became even more popular there. It was frequently applied in many street-front stores and even at the curbside.

9. Japanese Acupuncture

Acupuncture in Japan took several turns of its own, in addition to establishing the popularity of moxibustion. It paralleled the Chinese until the development of needle-less acupuncture (Shiatsu), which is now popular in the United States under the term *acupressure.* In many instances, acupressure can achieve acupuncture effects without the use of a needle—a decided advantage in our heavily needle-oriented society.

10. Ryodoraku

Ryodoraku is a particularly Japanese invention developed by a Japanese M.D., Dr. Nakatani. It is based on an electrical reading of the fingertips and toes, with the ancient meridians renumbered for simplicity. "Balancing the meridians" effects the cure of the disease that originally unbalanced them; because Dr. Nakatani is a licensed M.D., we could expect his theories, based on the action of the parasympathetic and sympathetic systems, to have some clinical validity.

11. Acupuncture in France

Acupuncture was introduced peremptorily in the ninth century. It was restarted in 1930 and developed successfully; today it is legally practiced only by licensed M.D.'s. In 1957, Dr. Paul Nogier, a Lyons neurophysiologist, was struck by some original ideas, which he coalesced into a modality called "Auriculotherapy." His theories of the homologous body points reproduced on the ear were later corroborated by the Chinese, and from this another ramification of acupuncture became established.

12. Reflexotherapy

Also in France, Dr. Henri Jarricot, working with neurological precision, developed a collection of acupuncture-like effects, which he grouped under the title of "Reflexotherapy." Both reflexotherapy and acupressure are closely allied to some facets of homeopathic and chiropractic medicine, and students of acupuncture should be the first to recognize this fact.

13. Acupuncture in England

In England, Sir Henry Head's theories seemed to explain many of the phenomena encountered in acupuncture, and a review of his material gave rise to several English schools of thought, among them Felix Mann's ideas on "short" and "long" reflexes.

14. Acupuncture in Russia

In Russia, a great deal of research was done on acupuncture; neuro-humoral and endocrine theories were added to the acupuncture horizon. The term Bio-energetics was used to group acupuncture with other phenomena such as parapsychology, Kirlian photography, and so on.

15. Acupuncture in the United States

Finally, in the United States, almost all practitioners have already practiced or performed an acupuncture-type procedure, under a different name of course. If they haven't, they have at least *heard* of the following:

a. "Dry Needling" of Trigger Points (Travell)
b. Electrical Anesthesia (Hardy, Fabian 1960) (Van Poznak, Artusio 1963)
c. Transcutaneous Stimulation (Shealy et al.)
d. Dorsal Column Stimulation (Sweet et al.)
e. Accelerated Wound Healing using electricity
f. Acupressure (see your local chiropractor)
g. Martial Arts (many points are identical with acupuncture points)

These American equivalents and derivatives of the ancient Oriental medical skill called acupuncture can be classified into the grouping called the acupuncture effect and must be considered to be part of the acupuncture panorama, regardless of what we may call it.

CHAPTER VI

PATHO-PHYSIOLOGY OF THE ACUPUNCTURE TREATMENT

"The Effects of Acupuncture on Cardio-Vascular and Nervous Systems"

Yoshiaki Omura, M.D., Sc.D.

Director of Medical Research, The Heart Disease Research Foundation, New York, N.Y., and Visiting Research Professor, Department of Electrical Engineering, Manhattan College, New York, N.Y., and Visiting Professor, University of Paris, Paris, France.

Introduction

Acupuncture, one branch of far eastern Oriental medicine, has been shown to be effective for many diseases and conditions.[1-18,21-26,32-38,54,74,77] Although acupuncture, just like any other medical treatment, has many limitations and advantages, the diseases or symptoms that can be helped effectively, but not in every case, by acupuncture include various pains such as migraine headaches, cramps, joint pain, musculo-skeletal pain, pain of the eye, trigerminal neuralgia, intercostal neuritis, shoulder pain, back pain, sciatic neuralgia, toothaches, pain due to certain types of herpes zoster, early stages of acute appendicitis due to the impact of fecal material, whiplash, tennis elbow, arthritis, gout, acute gallbladder due to stones, acute pain due to kidney stones, and intractable pain due to terminal cancer. Acupuncture has also been known to be effective for various problems, such as high blood pressure, blindness (due to circulatory disturbances in the eye-ground or brain),[13-15] deafness (particularly nerve deafness due to impaired circulation), Burger's disease, hemorrhoids, and diabetes.

Other symptoms or diseases which are helped by acupuncture are depressive states of schizophrenia, neurosis, insomnia and paralysis of the extremities, particularly those with spastic muscles (for instance, Dupruytren's contracture and torticollis),[13-15] facial nerve paralysis and facial muscle spasms, persistent hiccups, apoplexy (with spastic muscles), epilepsy, narrowing of the esophagus, neurogenic palpitations, anemia, spasms of the urinary bladder and urinary bladder paralysis, menstrual difficulty and excessive menstruation, post-partem hemmorhage, urticaria and otitis media. Acupuncture is also effective in treating hypersensitivity of the skin, accompanied by burning sensation and persistent pain which increases by friction of the skin, as well as in treating asthma and hay fever. Another interesting problem which is helped by acupuncture is obesity (some European classical acupuncture specialists claim acupuncture stimulates lipolysis), and withdrawal syndromes of the addiction to SNC depressants (narcotic analgesics such as opium and morphine, heroin, cocaine, barbiturates, alcohol, nicotine in tobacco, etc.) as well as some of the CNS stimulants.

If we classify all the diseases and symptoms which can be improved by acupuncture, we may be able to fit most of them into the following several categories, from their beneficial effects. The most significant and beneficial effects of acupuncture are:

1) relief from pain (analgesia)
2) relaxation of spastic muscles
3) relief of hypersensitivity of skin and mucous membrane to various factors
4) lowering of high blood pressure
5) improved circulation
6) stimulation of lipolysis
7) increase in immune responses and resistance to bacterial infections

However, as can be seen from the results of the author's research in the latter part of this article, this list itself, prepared by the author in the early part of 1972, is no longer sufficient to cover most of the beneficial effects of acupuncture. As a result, in June of 1973, the author expanded the beneficial effects of acupuncture into the following categories (some of these are closely interrelated).[13-15]

1) relief from pain (analgesia or hypoalgesia)

2) relaxation of spastic muscles
3) improved microcirculation (in local as well as distal parts of body by effectively induced vasodilation of capillaries and arterioles)
4) improved microcirculation in brain as a distal effect
5) lowering of high blood pressure
6) lowering of high blood lipid concentrations
7) relief from hypersensitivity of skin and mucous membrane to various factors
8) relief from mental depression (by mood elevation or euphoric effect) or hyperactive state or anxiety (by sedative or relaxation effect)
9) stimulation of anterior pituitary hormone release ACTH-like response by significant segmented neutrophilia and lymphcytopenia with or without eosinophilia)
10) increase in immune responses and resistance to bacterial infections
11) stimulation of lipolysis by secondary mechanism (primarily acupuncture appears to inhibit release of free fatty acid in albumin complex from adipose tissue)
12) some hypnotic effect (just as in any other treatment)

Often after patients have had acupuncture performed on them, regardless of what diseases the patients were treated for, the systolic blood pressure was lowered, and it was significantly lowered in those patients who had high blood pressure. There was some lowering of the diastolic blood pressure too. After receiving acupuncture, many patients also develop a feeling of various degrees of euphoria, sleepiness and a very comfortable sensation similar to the feeling one has immediately after taking a hot bath. However, these sensations are not always experienced in every patient. In acupuncture treatment, the most effective results are often obtained when insertion of the acupuncture needle is accompanied by heaviness or tingling or electric shock-like sensation which spreads to the distant parts of the body. If you place a needle at the *"tsu san-li"* (in Chinese, *ashi san-li* in Japanese) point (means literally three miles of leg and located on stomach meridian 36) of one of the legs, often the most effective beneficial results of lowering the blood pressure or relief of gastro-intestinal pain, are obtained when heaviness or tingling sensation or the electric shock-like sensations go down to the toe. This sensation is known as *"tei chi"* in Chinese (or *toku ki* in Japanese), which means "obtaining *qi* [*chi*]."

In Japan, they also describe this sensation as "*Hari* (needle) *no* (of) *hibiki* (echo)" which means echo of acupuncture.[9-10] Whenever you have this "*hibiki*," the result is often remarkable. Whenever acupuncture produces relief of pain or relaxation of spastic muscles, various degrees of warm sensation develop around the area where acupuncture was given. When the sensation of warmness is felt, the increase in the various degree of skin temperature can be measured with a thermister thermometer or by the appearance of various colors of liquid crystal or by infra-red thermography.

These clinical findings, which we often observed, indicated that at least both the circulatory system (including the lymph system) and the nervous system must be involved in the genesis of beneficial acupuncture effects. Thus, we have been very much interested in finding out the effects of acupuncture on peripheral circulation, brain circulation, electrocardiogram, heart sound and temperature as well as the effects of acupuncture on the nervous system, electroencephalograms, somato-sensory evoked potentials, pain thresholds, particularly on the motor-nerve conduction velocity and sensory nerve conduction velocity, since the phenomena of "*toku-ki*" is one of the results of the stimulation of the sensory nerve which can be felt by the patient as a spreading sensation to the distant parts of the body. "*Toku-ki*" is also often accompanied by stimulation of the motor nerves.

Anatomical Considerations of Epidermis, Dermis, Subcutaneous Tissue and Their Relationship to Acupuncture Needles:

As soon as the acupuncture needle penetrates the skin, depending upon the anatomical structures of the skin, the patient will feel various degrees of pain sensation, since most of the skin has many pain sensitive nerve endings in two different forms: either as small-diametered naked unmyelinated nerve endings of C-fibers or various forms of myelinated nerve endings of A-group delta fibers. These fibers are mainly concentrated just in the dermis (see Figure in "Pain: Morphologic Aspects" by M. R. Millers in the book *New Concepts in Pain and Its Clinical Management*, edited by E. L. Way and its modified diagram in ref. 13-15,74,77). As soon as the needle is inserted into the skin, whether the patient feels pain depends upon whether the acupuncture needle directly hit or indirectly irritated the nerve ending which transmits the pain sensation. Even if the pain-sensitive nerve endings are irritated by the acupuncture needle, if simultaneously the patient's attention is directed to some other part of the body, or penetration is done very quickly, the immediate pain sensation is often unnoticed by the patient. Since most of the nerve endings, which transmit the pain sensation, such as unmyelinated C-fibers or myelinated A-group delta fingers, are located mainly in the dermis (although some of the unmyelinated C-fibers can also be found around the basal cell layer of the epidermal tissue), which is located a short distance away from the surface of the skin, these small diametered nerve fibers' nerve endings are responsible for the pain sensation. The rest of the large diametered myelinated nerve endings is also a short distance away from the skin, mainly in the dermis and scattered at the subcutaneous tissue, where there are networks of capillaries and lymph channels. Therefore, the pain which may accompany surgery usually comes at the moment incision of the dermis is made, while incision of the subcutaneous tissue is associated with very little pain sensation. The degree of the pain sensation depends not only upon the location of the skin hit by the acupuncture needle, but also by the type of acupuncture needle used. The larger the acupuncture needle, the greater the chance that there will be pain sensation at the time of penetration of needle into the skin. In general, the smaller the needle, the less the pain sensation. However, the tip of the needle is another important factor in the presence or absence of pain sensation. If the tip has a sharp point, you will have a relatively smaller amount of pain than with an acupuncture needle that has a deformity at the tip. Such abnormalities can be detected easily by microscopic examination. If one compares the typical examples of acupuncture needles with hypodermic needles, acupuncture needles with fancy handles and diameters of 0.279 mm are typical examples of acupuncture needles produced in China, and the acupuncture needle with a small diameter of 0.254 is a typical example of Japanese acupuncture needles. All of these acupuncture needles can fit into the lumen of the hypodermic needle, gauge no. 25.

If one compares critically the damage of the tissue with the insertion of hypodermic needle, one will find that the acupuncture needle is much safer than the hypodermic needle, since the hypodermic needle has a much larger diameter but also has a sharp cutting edge which can destroy the tissue, while the acupuncture needle penetrates the tissue but does much less damage. Once the acupuncture needle punctures the skin, the first sensation the patient experiences will be the various degrees of pain sensation, initiating at the point the needle is inserted and then followed by the following series of consecutive changes: [13–15,24–29,39–67,74–77]

1) a rather sharp pain (mainly due to the stimulation of A-group delta fibers)
2) soreness characterized by a dull pain (due to the stimulation of C-fibers)
3) heaviness (due to the stimulation of pressure sensitive corpuscles)
4) swelling (due to interference of microcirculatory system and increased permeability)
5) a reddish corona around the acupuncture needle insertion point (due to local vasodilation of capillaries and arterioles)
6) a warm sensation develops around the needle point (due to the improvement in microcirculation)
7) continued manipulation of the needle eventually produces an increased pain threshold or numbness (analgesia or hypoalgesia effect)
8) by further continuous manipulation of the needle (45-60 min.) the numbness (local analgesic effect) will spread to distal area gradually along certain areas of the body or in some cases suddenly appear in certain parts of the distal part of the body and can be used as one means of producing analgesia required for surgical operations.

If you look at the skin around the acupunctured point you will see either the homogenous reddish corona due to the arteriolar and capillary dilations, or you will see a reddish star or netlike appearance due to the microhermorrhages.

Effects of Acupuncture on the Circulatory System

Non-invasive Method of Studying the Effects of Acupuncture on Peripheral and Brain Circulations:

Any study to measure the effects of acupuncture must be performed with non-invasive methods, since introduction of any needle into the body is considered to be a type of acupuncture. As a non-invasive means of studying the effects of acupuncture, in addition to electro-cardiogram, heart sound recording, the most useful information can be obtained by measuring the blood pressure pulse wave pattern changes. The analysis of this will give us a great deal of useful information. One of the simplest means of studying the blood pressure pulse wave patterns is the indirect method of using the photoelectric plethysmographic (PEPG) sensor. Presently the most widely used photoelectric plethysmographic method is the transmission type, in which one must place a part of the body between the light source and photoelectric detector. Therefore, the use of the transmission type photoelectric plethysmographic method is limited to the fingers, earlobes, or penis, and for convenience the fingers are most often used. However, according to our study, we found the amount of intensity of light needed to produce a significantly detectable change through the body tissue is very high, and it increases the temperature of the skin. As a result the circulatory state of the area of the body through which the light passes is considerably and artificially changed. Therefore, an accurate response cannot be measured by the transmission type PEPG sensor. Secondly, in the use of the patients' fingers, the circulation of both sides of the finger is quite different and the tissue between the front and back of the finger has different distributions of capillary networks and arterioles. Thus, any measurement by the transmission type photoelectric plethysmographic sensors can be assumed to be inaccurate, and to confirm this suspicion we did a series of tests. In addition, most of the sensors used for the transmission type photoelectric plethysmography had considerably longer time constants in comparison to the claims of the manufacturers. Many of them had a time constant of more than 50 milliseconds which means that any phenomenon occurring for less than 50 milliseconds was deformed or completely disappeared, due to poor frequency response of the detector side of the sensor. To eliminate these difficulties, the author developed during the period 1969-1971, an ultra-miniature, reflection type, photoelectric plethysmographic sensor by which we were able to eliminate all of the currently existing difficulties found with the transmission type sensor. The frequency response is less than 0.2 milliseconds and the size is less than a few hundredths of the size of transmission type photoelectric plethymographic sensor unit. Because of its excellent frequency response and small size with minimum artifact, we have been able to measure the various states of the blood circulation from practically any part of the body surface of a human being. For instance, using this sensor we also found that we can measure the circulatory states at the tip of the nose, at the cheek, chin, forehead, neck, chest, abdomen, nail head, palm of the hand, toe, etc. While measuring the circulation at different parts of the body surface, we noticed striking differences in the pattern obtained at certain parts of the forehead. After a series of studies we confirmed that the circulation measured with our sensors at certain parts of the forehead represented the brain circulation coming from the supra-orbital artery, which is a branch of the ophthalmic artery, which is in turn a major branch of the internal carotid artery, that is a major artery of the brain. Thus we were able to find that in a normal person, between 65 and 95 percent of the blood circulation at certain parts of the forehead is due to brain circulation, and in a majority of people the blood circulation at certain parts of the forehead is supplied more than 85 percent by the supra-orbital artery alone. Therefore, we established one of the most simple non-traumatic means of studying the brain circulation known, without sticking a needle into the body, but simply by placing our own improved reflection type photoelectric plethysmographic sensor at the area where the blood supplies are coming mainly from the supra-orbital artery. Using this technique of studying the peripheral circulation and brain circulation, we did a series of experiments on the making of differential diagnoses on patients who have a variety of cardiovascular diseases. Some of these results were reported in the International Congress of Pharmacology, held in San Francisco, in July 1972.[19,20] Using this new technique, we were able to make a differential diagnosis of at least 17 different abnormal cardiovascular states. To insure the accuracy of such a simple useful technique, we also measured electro-cardiograms and heart sound simultaneously. Thus whenever the diagnosis by PEPG wave pattern alone is suspicious, but all three parameters taken simultaneously indicate one identical diagnosis, one has an absolute diagnosis, which is obtained entirely by non-traumatic means.

Thus, we are interested in studying the effect of acupuncture on cardiovascular systems by our technique of studying the peripheral and brain circulations, using our improved sensor "ultra miniature reflection type photoelectric plethysmographic sensor with short response time."

The Effect of Acupuncture on Peripheral and Brain Circulation:

By April 1972, using our improved ultra-miniature reflection-type photoelectric sensor with a very short response time,[19,20] we repeatedly measured consecutively changing phases of circulatory response to the insertion and manipulation of the acupuncture needles into the body, and the author classified these changes into the following three consecutive phases:[12,15-22,24-55,60-75,77]

1) *1st Phase:* Vaso-constriction—usually lasts 15-30 sec.
2) *2nd Phase:* Quasi-control site—usually lasts 10 sec.-2 min.

3) *3rd Phase:* Vaso-dilation—usually lasts 2 min.-2 or 3 weeks

This was observed in more than 50% of the 208 cases examined by the end of 1972 and not only in the local area where acupuncture was performed, but often in distant areas, including brain circulation. We detected distinctive vaso-dilation during or following acupuncture, with blood pressure often going down significantly in those with high blood pressure or decreasing slightly in those who had near normal blood pressure. Whenever acupuncture produced the immediate significant relief of pain or relaxation of spastic muscles, we were almost always able to measure significant vaso-dilation (of capillaries and arterioles) of not only the local area but also vaso-dilation of distal areas of the body including brain, accompanied by a decrease in blood pressure and an increase in local temperature due to improved micro circulation. Immediately following the relief of pain or relaxation of muscle from the shoulder, arm, or hand, the maximum grasping force of the affected hand often increases significantly whenever the grasping force before acupuncture is markedly diminished, although there are exceptions. Whenever significant improvement in brain circulation is observed, the patient becomes euphoric and sometimes is so relaxed and comfortable that he often wants to take a nap. Therefore, all our studies indicate that development of significant vaso-dilation of capillaries and arterioles is essential for obtaining relief of pain and relaxation of spastic muscles. Whenever the patient experienced prolonged pain sensation after acupuncture, we found unusually prolonged vaso-constriction following acupuncture. This was seen relatively often among people who had severe asthma and various allergies simultaneously. Vaso-constriction is also observed frequently when acupuncture is performed above the neck, especially at the head in these patients.

Effect of Acupuncture on High Blood Pressure:

The most effective generalized vaso-dilation was observed when acupuncture was given at "*tsu san-li*" (*ashi san-li* in Japanese) points (stomach 36) of the legs. The vaso-dilation effect was often extended to many distal parts of the body, including the brain. The maximum effect was observed whenever "*toku-ki*" was experienced by inserting the needle in a rather localized certain area near the surface of the tibial bone facing the fibular bone. For instance, a 2-4-minute continuous manipulation of "*tsu san-li*" point of the left leg alone reduced blood pressure from 200/110 mmHg to 150/95 mmHg which lasted for six days. However, if manipulation of the needle is not done properly so that it creates considerable intense prolonged pain consistently for more than 30 sec.-few min., transitionally the blood pressure may go up significantly. Therefore, proper experience and basic knowledge in treating very high blood pressure is essential. Whenever acupuncture was effective in reducing high blood pressure, we also found significant decreases (often 30-60% decrease) in the serum concentration of triglyceride, and phospholipid (measured in form of lecithin) and less significant decreases (10-30% decrease) in cholesterol, particularly in those people who have had a high concentration of these components before acupuncture. Sometimes the effects on blood chemistry lasted for more than ten days.

Even without using acupuncture needles, by simply pressing the same acupuncture point very hard with the finger tip, similar but less effective results can be obtained in many patients, especially when heaviness or dull pain or electric shock-like or tingling sensations propagate to distal parts and go down to the toe. Other points (more correctly, areas) effective in lowering high blood pressure were found accidentally. Whenever we treated middle-aged or elderly patients for shoulder pains or tightness of the shoulder muscle, in those who happened to have high blood pressure, the blood pressure was often decreased after acupuncture, with similar changes in blood chemistry. Also, a similar phenomenon was observed in patients who had combined shoulder and neck pain, and shoulder and neck muscle tightness.

Having obtained results that are quite different from our findings, a well-known French acupuncture specialist, Dr. Nguyen Van Nghi, reported during an acupuncture seminar held in Connecticut in June of 1972, that the best results in lowering blood pressure could be obtained with acupuncture administered on several points on the front and back of the chest on the hypersensitive patient. The maximum decrease he obtained was 10-15 mmHg, which occurred within one hour after acupuncture was performed on these several points of the body, with pressure returning to its original state within 15 hours, which was shown with only Data of Blood Pressure plotting. Dr. Van Nghi explained the mechanism for lowering blood pressure with the classical Chinese meridian theory and the classical concept of the so-called flow of "energy." However, after learning of the results of this author's intensive basic research on human beings, he was kind enough to accept the author's findings and mention in subsequent talks in the same meeting that the *"tsu san-li"* points are more effective in lowering high blood pressure than many other acupuncture points. He promptly provided his own interpretation to explain why acupuncture administered to the *"tsu san-li"* points is so effective in lowering high blood pressure using classical Chinese acupuncture theory.

During the same meeting, Dr. Felix Mann, president of the British Acupuncture Society, was honest enough to tell me that acupuncture given at the *"tsu san-li"* points usually did not produce any significant lowering effect for high blood pressure, but he also informed this author that he usually manipulated the acupuncture needles for only about 25 seconds although occasionally up to one minute or more. In fact, many acupuncture specialists twirl the needles for a rather short period of time and then leave the needle in the body tissue for somewhere between 5 to 30 minutes for treating patients with various symptoms. Although these examples of the experiences of others are completely contradictory in appearance to what the author has found, these differences can be explained by the author's finding that maximum generalized vaso-dilation is usually obtained when manual twirling is given properly and continued for at least 1 to 2 minutes, often for 2 minutes or even longer depending upon individual patients as well as the technique and the length of the needle inserted below skin, at a rate of twirling of 2-4 seconds. Generalized vaso-dilation can also be obtained by widely used classical acupuncture technique too, but this is often insignificant. On the other hand, without accurate monitoring set up, occasionally observed undesirable unsually strong prolonged vaso-constriction in those who were allergic to many substances can be minimized as long as the manipulation is limited to less than 25 seconds. Since the author made known his research findings in 1972, many people in various parts of the world have begun to recognize the advantage of the prolonged manipulation compared with the result obtained simply by leaving the needle in the body tissue without much twirling.

In early 1972 Chinese and Japanese literature on the treatment of high blood presure with acupuncture[1, 18-25-26-32, 38-67, 69] indicated that there were at least ten pairs of classical acupuncture points (four pairs on the ear) and a few on the conception and governing vessels known to be effective in treating high blood pressure, among them the *"tsu san-li"* points of both legs which are included as supplemental rather than as points of primary importance. The author's comparative studies with hypertensive patients on the effectiveness of acupuncture on the basis of measured degrees of acupuncture induced generalized vaso-dilation (mainly of the capillaries and arterioles) indicates that most of the so-called acupuncture points of primary importance in lowering high blood pressure are not as effective as the "*tsu san-li*" points in inducing generalized vaso-dilation and consequently not as effective in lowering high blood pressure. Details of the technique used to obtain maximum generalized vaso-dilation will be described in the forthcoming books of the author.

Effects of Acupuncture on Low Blood Pressure:

In early 1972, I was very much interested in finding out whether or not acupuncture could possibly reduce blood pressure to a seriously low level in people who had already very low blood pressure. We studied both 5 adult patients who had very low systolic blood pressure of less than 100 mmHg and were doing normal work and more than 20 adults who had systolic blood pressure of less than 110 mmHg. To our surprise, acupuncture usually did not lower the blood pressure significantly in those patients, but we often saw a slight increase in the systolic blood pressure. Therefore, generally speaking, proper use of acupuncture can control abnormal blood pressure level to the optimal range. For instance, some points in the face (*jin-chu* in Japanese, in Chinese *lun chung* governing vessel 26) or in the foot (kidney 1) are very effective in raising blood pressure in those patients whose blood pressure becomes acutely low. However, a great amount of interesting research remains to be investigated in this area, in those who have very low blood pressure. Whenever acupuncture produces relief of pain or relaxation of spastic muscles in extremities, significant vaso-dilation of the arterioles and capillaries can be found around the local area, along with warm sensation felt by the patient and increase in temperature. Following relief of pain from shoulder or arm or hand, grasping force of the affected hand often increases significantly. However, when acupuncture is performed on the extremities of the patients with low blood pressure, the distal effect on the brain circulation is often not significant.

Effects of Acupuncture on the Electrocardiogram and Heart Sound:

In spite of the fact that the beneficial effects of acupuncture such as relief of pain, or relaxation of spastic muscles, are almost always accompanied by a significant amount of vaso-dilation of the arterioles and capillaries not only in the area where acupuncture is performed but also in the distal areas of the body, one might think there should be significant changes in the electrocardiogram and heart sound. However, in the majority of cases, the changes in the electrocardiogram and heart sound are not significant, although often a slight increase in heart beat is observed with a slight decrease in the Q-T interval. The most significant changes we encountered were those found in the patients who had fainting spells. In these people, usually heart rate diminished, often accompanied with prolongation of each wave of the electrocardiogram. As I described previously, these people had striking increases in conduction velocity of both motor and sensory nerves and diminished brain circulation. The detailed analysis of the effect of acupuncture on EEG and heart sound will be published by the author elsewhere.

The Effects of Acupuncture on the Blood:

1) Effects of acupuncture on the red blood cells and white blood cells and cell differentials:

In general, it has been believed that red blood cells often increase and there should be a signficant increase in the white blood cell count. According to our study this does not always occur. As a matter of fact, sometimes there is a decrease in the number of both red and white cells. When acupuncture manipulation (each lasting 2-4 min. continuously) was performed on more than five or ten points, more than 50 percent of patients developed a degree of increase in the white blood cell count. However, the most significant changes in the differential of the white blood cells were frequently observed in a majority of the cases of patients who received acupuncture treatment, particularly within 24 hours after receiving acupuncture. The largest changes are usually observed as an increase in the percentage of the segmented neutrophiles of the white blood cells. Often the segmented neutrophiles increase 20-50 percent, and the percentage of the lymphocytes decreases significantly with or without increase in eosinophilic cells. However, these changes in white cell differentials are expected since acupuncture is a (mechanical) injury to the body tissues which is followed by the typical inflammatory process.[55,58]

2) Effects of acupuncture on blood chemistry:

The most significant and interesting changes in blood chemistry observed by the author in early 1972 were the concentrations of serum triglycerides, phospholipids, and cholesterol. In those who have high blood pressure, often there was also an increased concentration of some or all of these three components of blood chemistry. Whenever we performed acupuncture, we observed a significant decrease (often 30-60% decrease) in the concentration of triglycerides, phospholipids and less significant decrease (10-30%) in cholesterol after acupuncture. Whenever significant vaso-dilation was observed with our technique, it was usually accompanied by a decrease in blood pressure (when pre-acupuncture blood pressure was very high or slightly above normal) and these changes in blood chemistry. Therefore, since more than 10% of the population of the United States is believed to have high blood pressure and the number of treatments for this is limited, the author's findings in blood chemistry as well as blood pressure decrease may provide another form of possible treatment and may have important clinical application worthy of further investigation. CPK often increased after acupuncture up to 150% increase, but frequently its increase did not exceed more than 80%, SGOT and LDH often increased slightly but they were often insignificant. In a majority of cases, glucose increased 15-35%, but in less than 10% of the cases, increase of glucose went up to +120%. In less than 25% of the cases, serum glucose concentration diminished but the range of the decreases were within -30%. Significant increases (more than 15%) in serum glucose were also often associated with the appearance of generalized vaso-dilation of capillaries and arterioles.

The most significant blood chemistry change after acupuncture was in the triglycerides and phospholipids. These components went down significantly, with sometimes more than 50% decreases accompanied by the significant decrease in serum lipo-proteins such as pre-B-lipoprotein. Another interesting change found by the author through the study of a series of electrophoresis of serum proteins: after acupuncture in some cases there was very slow but significant increase in the gamma-globulin fraction of serum protein. This increase in serum globulin concentration may be one of the major reasons for the well-known fact that acupuncture increases the resistance to infectious disease and may enhance the immune response to produce sufficient antibodies. The changes in electrolytes were usually insignificant. Serotonin often increased slightly (usually within +40%), particularly when electra-acupuncture is given through the part of the head. Concentration of serotonin in the jugular vein is slightly higher than in the brachial vein. This may be the result of significant increase in serotonin in certain parts of the brain. Details of other blood chemistry changes will be discussed elsewhere.

The Effect of Acupuncture on the Nervous System:[12,15-39,54-77-79]

The most effective result of acupuncture is often seen after having the sensation of *"toku-ki,"* which can be interpreted as a stimulation of the sensory nerve fibers, often along with stimulation of the motor nerve fibers. It seems to me that, in addition to the circulatory system (including the lymph system), the nervous system is also closely involved in obtaining the beneficial effects of acupuncture. Therefore, most of the patients whom we have accepted as experimental subjects for our research have had both motor nerve and sensory nerve conduction velocities as well as other parameters related to the nervous system examined before and after acupuncture, in addition to studies on the circulatory system.

1) Effects of acupuncture on motor nerve conduction velocity:

Motor nerve conduction velocities were measured by electrical simulation of various peripheral nerves, non-invasively, from the outside of the skin at various parts of the body's surface. However, for the sake of simplicity, we often used the ulnar nerves of both the right and left hands. We stimulated the ulnar nerve at the elbow, with the square-wave electrical pulse generator, and an electromyogram generated by the corresponding muscle fibers measured the response at the corresponding part of the palm of the hand. The proper stimulation of the nerve was identifiable by the visible flexing of the fourth and fifth fingers. The measurement of the electromyogram was done with the tektronix D.C. Dual beam oscilloscope at the sensitivity of 0.2 millivolt/cm-1.0 millivolt/cm. with a sweep of 2 milliseconds/cm-5 milliseconds/cm. Stimulation of the ulnar nerve was made at one or two more points along the ulnar nerve in addition to the one at the elbow.

In the same person conduction velocities are usually quite consistent and their daily variations were within 5%. Normal conduction velocities before acupuncture in the majority of the people were between 65 m/sec.-80 m/sec. Two patients had a conduction velocity before acupuncture of more than 90 m/sec. In these two cases, acupuncture in a certain part of the back produced fainting, with decreased heart rate and significant vaso-constriction in the brain. This is one of the few cases where the patients experienced fainting.

Of the other extreme cases we observed, we found a few patients with extremely low conduction velocities. In these cases we found that one person had been drinking alcohol intensely before we took the measurement. In another case the person had been drinking plus regularly using Librium. After repeating the tests without the patient taking alcohol, we still found that a low conduction velocity of less than 55 m/sec. persisted until the Librium was discontinued. In this last case the person took Librium regularly and her conduction velocity was less than 60 m/sec.

All of these problems were not stated by the patients, even when asked if they were using liquor or sedatives, until the conduction velocity was shown to be so low that either something was wrong with them or else they were taking medication which was slowing down the conduction velocity.

When acupuncture was given outside of the ulnar nerve for a period of more than 3-4 min., there was no significant change observed in conduction velocity of the ulnar nerve between the point of electrical stimulation and wrist. When acupuncture is given near the ulnar nerve or any other nerve fibers, there is always some degree of decrease of conduction velocity in the small part of the nerve fibers located within about 5-10 mm from the acupunctured loci. But there were no significant changes in conduction velocities of the rest of the motor nerve fibers. Even after 15 minutes of continuous manipulation of the needle, the decrease in conduction velocity was usually very small. The maximum decrease in conduction velocity was about 25%. However, manipulation of less than 5 minutes usually produced less than 10% decrease in conduction velocity. Threshold stimulation (for the given period pulse duration of 0.1-0.5 m/sec.) for square-wave electric impulse is often enhanced up to 250% following the administration of acupuncture of 2-4 min. at the same area where electrical stimulation was applied non-invasively from the surface of the skin.

2) Effects of acupuncture on sensory nerve conduction velocity:

Although the maximum of certain potentials of the sensory nerve fiber of the ulnar nerve is detectable from the body surface above the nerve, it is usually much less than 10 microvolts and is buried in large random noises. Because of noise interference, unless the transient signal averaging method is used, it is difficult to observe the electrograms of nerve fibers *in situ* clearly from the body surface. However, such a transient signal averaging device is expensive and not convenient for this purpose. We used instead a simpler and less expensive method, the mono-synaptic reflex pathway of the spinal cord. Namely, we used the Hoffman reflex (H-reflex). Using the same set-up as the motor nerve conduction velocity measurement at a certain stimulation voltage given at the sensory nerve, the excitation of the sensory nerve fibers will be created. Propagation of such an electric impulse goes to the dorsal column of the spinal cord. Then, through one synapse at the spinal cord, the impulse goes to the same muscle where one is measuring the electro-myogram, for measurement of the motor nerve conduction velocity. Thus, by stimulation of certain points of the ulnar nerve, and measurement of the electro-myogram potentials due to direct stimulation of the motor nerves innervating the responsible muscle fibers for the recorded EMG. Then around 50 milliseconds later, we can observe a small second electro-myogram due to the H-reflex. By repeating similar measurements through stimulation of an additional one or two points of the ulnar nerve, we can estimate the conduction velocity of the sensory nerve fiber. Such a measurement shows that an average conduction velocity of the sensory nerve fibers is about 10 meters less than the motor nerve fibers. The effects of acupuncture are quite similar to those found in the motor nerve fiber conduction velocity of the same person.

3) Effects of acupuncture on the electroencephalograms (EEGs):

Although we have not done any intensive study on this subject before the end of 1972, we have made recordings of EEGs on about 15 patients, before and after acupuncture. These have shown that whenever we detected insignificant vaso-dilation of capillaries and arterioles in the brain, significant bursting of alpha waves has predominantly appeared for a period of less than 15 min.; the patients are relaxed and comfortable, without many worries or fears, and often become euphoric for much longer time durations—not only individuals without psychiatric diseases, but also some with mental depression and schizophrenia. Since 1973, with Professor Andre Sourailac, M.D., Sc.D., Director and Chairman of the Dept. of Psycho-physiology and his associates Noah Hardy and others, and Professor G. Nahas and his associates at the Institute of Anesthesiology of the University of Paris VI (part of the Old

Sorbonne), the author began collaborative research on the effects of acupuncture on EEGs of psychiatric patients and normal individuals to evaluate the author's theory that, through leaky cell membranes due to mechanical agitations or stimulations by acupuncture or shiatsu or contractions of muscles by electrical stimulations, certain chemical substances, including enzymes and some of the prostaglandins, are released from the interior of the cells to the surrounding area and go to the circulatory system and are carried to distal parts of the body and influence both the circulatory and nervous systems at the distal parts of the body, and that the amounts of the released substances are proportional to the numbers of the mechanically stimulated cells. The time required for the striking bursting appearance of alpha waves following the acupuncture given at different parts of the body of the same subject indicated that the further the distance between brain and acupunctured area, the longer the time required. This finding indirectly supported the author's hypothesis, namely "Circulatory-Nervous Systems' Multi-parameter Chemo-humor-neural Interactions Theory" with additional introduction of the concept of functional unit of "Neuro-Musculo-Vascular Unit" rather than the widely used narrow concept of "Neuro-Muscular Unit."

The Effect of Acupuncture on the Digestive System:

Stimulation of sympathetic and parasympathetic nerves by acupuncture can change the peristalsis of the stomach, by which it can influence the amount of secretion of the digestive juices, particularly that of hydro-chloric acid. For instance, using a rabbit, dogs or humans, the effects of acupuncture on "*tsu san-li*" points can be demonstrated as a decrease in peristalsis of the stomach, and sometimes other parts of the G.I. system, particularly when the peristalsis is abnormally enhanced. One of the most convenient clinical applications is the use of the "*tsu san-li*" points even without using the needle. Various kinds of abdominal pain, including pain due to the early stage of acute appendicitis where the muscle wall of the appendix is irritated by the impact of fecal material and the muscles of the appendix are spastic, which in turn impairs the circulation and reduces the resistance to bacterial infection, can often be reduced or eliminated by simply pressing the acupuncture point with the finger tip (= "*Shiatsu*" in Japanese). However, if the appendicitis is already advanced, one should not waste time with this method. If the cause of such a pain remains in the gastro-intestinal system, the pain eventually will recur, but if the cause of the pain is removed, the relief from the pain remains for a long period of time. In short, without using needles, "*Shiatsu*" alone at "*tsu san-li*" is often effective in reducing acute G.I. pain.

The Effect of Acupuncture on the Endocrine System:

When the acupuncture produces persistent vaso-constriction, accompanied by severe pain, or simply produces a severe pain for a prolonged period of more than 10 or 20 seconds, secretion of the catecholamimes often increases. Usually secretion of adrenalin significantly increases by persistent pain sensation, created by acupuncture or during acupuncture, but when the pain disappears, such a secretion returns to normal. Increased secretion of adrenalin has further contributed to the vaso-constriction and enhances the blood pressure and increases the heart rate. However, when acupuncture is done properly, in the majority of the patients, increase in blood pressure and increase in the heart rate are not significant. Even if they were significant, usually they would not last for more than 30 seconds. The phenomenon of significant segmented neutrophilia and lymphocytopenia with or without eosinophilia, frequently found in our studies after acupuncture, resembles the effects of ACTH administration in individuals with normal functions of anterior pituitary gland and adrenal cortex. This may be due to the stimulation of the anterior pituitary gland following the release of certain chemical substances from the interior of cells surrounding the acupunctured area. The effects on the other hormones will be reported elsewhere.

The Effects of Acupuncture on the Respiratory System:

Acupuncture given at the "*hoku*" points (large intestine 4) of one of the hands or "Sudden Heaven" (conception vessel 22) induced significant improvement, up to 150%, in the parameters of the respiratory function examined by the photographic recording of a spirostat in those who are suffering from the paralysis of extremities with or without difficulty in breathing, due to various diseases such as poliomyelitis, multiple sclerosis, amyotrophic lateral sclerosis, as well as in those patients with asthma. The most frequent improvement is between +10-60% which was seen often immediately after acupuncture in those who have diminished respiratory functions. Similar improvement in respiratory function was obtained by effectively applied "*Shiatsu*" on these acupuncture loci. The most useful clinical application of acupuncture given at the "*hoku*" points of the hands is that an asthma attack can often be eliminated. However, effectively giving finger pressure alone without using any needles on these acupuncture loci also eliminated asthma attack. The author has worked with many patients who have suffered from frequent attacks of asthma for many years (some of them for more than 35 years) on whom strong finger pressure on one of the above-described, as well as a few other points, not only abolished the attack within five minutes, but also diminished markedly the intensity and frequency of asthma attacks. In 1972 the author speculated that mechanical stimulation of the cells releases certain chemical substances, including some of the prostaglandins which improve microcirculation of the transitionally impaired micro-circulatory networks of lungs as well as the spastic bronchial muscles. Since most of the anti-asthmatic agents are B-adrenergic receptor stimulants, they not only relax the spastic bronchial muscles, but also induce the undesirable effect of increasing heart rate and increasing the contractile force of the heart by the undesirable increase in the myocardial consumption of 0_2. Therefore, such a non-invasive method which eliminates the use of drugs has considerable clinical value in the treatment of asthma. Since the author first reported this method at lectures and symposiums in the United States and at many universities in Europe in mid-1972, it has now been used clinically by many people with considerable success.

The Effect of the Hypnotic Factor on Acupuncture Treatment:

Many distinguished physicians have claimed, formally or informally, that the beneficial effects of acupuncture are to a great extent due to hypnotic factors which are produced by the acupuncturist consciously or unconsciously. One of the first successful surgical operations employing acupuncture analgesia in the United States was a skin graft operation performed by Dr. G. Ephron at the university hospital of Albert Einstein College of Medicine to cover a large ulcerated leg. Acupuncture analgesia was administered by Dr. Frank Z. Warren, Dr. Pang L. Man and Dr. Yoshiaki Omura by combined use of electroacupuncture and manual acupuncture under the direct supervision of Dr. Louis R. Orkin,

Professor and Chairman of the Department of Anesthesiology of Albert Einstein College of Medicine. A leading neuro-physiologist, Dr. Vernon B. Mountcastle, Professor and Chairman of the Department of Physiology at John Hopkins University Medical School, stated that he believed that the effects of acupuncture in this operation were "specious" (see "Acupuncture Is Used To Anesthesize a Patient Here," *N.Y. Times*, Tues., May 30, 1972, p. 24). The author, knowing the careful work of Dr. Mountcastle, feels that he meant to say that "acupuncture anesthesia" rather than "acupuncture analgesia" is specious, because in 1972 many people incorrectly used the phrase "acupuncture anesthesia" instead of "acupuncture analgesia" or more correctly "acupuncture hypo-algesia" in spite of the fact that acupuncture reduces pain sensations and relaxes spastic muscles while the patient is completely awake and conscious. (See also *N.Y. Post*, Tues., May 30, 1972, "First Acupuncture Surgery Here a Success.")

Dr. Herbert Spiegel, the renowned medical hypnotist, and Clinical Associate Professor of Psychiatry at Columbia University, has repeatedly emphasized that acupuncture is a "ritualistic form of hypnosis." There are a few influential well-known professors of anesthesiology in the U.S. who have ideas similar to those of Dr. Spiegel, but the demonstration of the beneficial effects of acupuncture which cannot be accounted for by hypnosis alone has made them change some of their feelings about acupuncture.

To evaluate the effect of hypnosis, the author began to use the "Eye Roll Test"[70] which is the simplest and quickest method of evaluating the hypnotizability of the human subject. It was first reported by Dr. Spiegel in 1970 (as one part of his more complete hypnotic induction profile) and was derived from an analysis of 2,000 consecutive cases in which he used the same trance induction procedure. This "Eye Roll" sign predicts hypnotizability in three out of four cases, and the higher the eye roll measured on a scale of 0 to 4, the higher the trance capacity to be expected. Since the end of 1972, the author began to use this criteria as part of the examination of all patients before administering acupuncture, but results indicate that the degree of beneficial effects produced by acupuncture and the degree of hypnotizability was not proportional, that is, some of those who showed a high susceptibility to hypnosis obtained very little beneficial effects of acupuncture, while others with a low hypnotizability rating developed significant improvement of their symptoms. The most striking fact is that among those who scored low on the hypnotizability from symptoms in more than 70 percent of the cases, most of which were accompanied by generalized vaso-dilation, CBC and blood chemistry changes. In mid-1973, when the author tried to evaluate the meaning of the currently used concept that hypnosis has nothing to do with sleep but is an intensive form of mental concentration, he realized that some of the patients in his previous study who had a diminished brain micro-circulation with diminished ability to concentrate or memorize and a high degree of irritability or insomnia before acupuncture often experienced improved brain micro-circulation strikingly after acupuncture with concomitant improvement in memory and ability to concentrate and other symptoms. The author began to use the "Eye Roll Test" both before and after acupuncture and in some cases found increases in the test score after acupuncture. Therefore, while there is some hypnotic factor involved before acupuncture just as in any modality of medical treatment, particularly when the patient has confidence in both the physician and the treatment, it is not a major factor in producing acupuncture effects. Yet, in those who develop increased "Eye Roll Test" scores after acupuncture, hypnosis may play some important role in attaining or self-evaluating the beneficial effects of acupuncture in some cases.

Discussion and Summary

To explain the known clinically observed phenomenon associated with acupuncture, one must first recognize that both the circulatory and the nervous systems are simultaneously affected. Thus, it is imperative to study the effects of acupuncture on both the cardio-vascular and nervous systems at the same time, since study of only one part of the phenomena will not reveal the mutually related complex electrophysiological as well as biochemical interactions between the circulatory and nervous systems. Therefore, the author's research has been concentrated on both the circulatory and nervous systems.

Study of one patient usually requires somewhere between three to nine hours (including our routine pre- and post-acupuncture physical examination and eye roll test to evaluate hypnotizability, each of which requires about 30-60 mins.) of continuous monitoring of the various parameters depending upon the relative completeness or partiality of study and sometimes more than 10 rolls of Polaroid film for the recording of the parameters for our relatively complete study. More than 30 different blood chemistries were measured within 24 hours before, immediately after, and within 24 hours after acupuncture, then again one and two weeks after acupuncture treatment, for a total of five times. However, because of the sizable expense involved in these tests we eventually settled for the basic requirement that the patient undergo blood chemistry tests within 24 hours before, within 24 hours after and one week after acupuncture treatment. Another reason for eliminating the test immediately after acupuncture is that usually we found no significant change in blood chemistry and CBC immediately after and within three hours after acupuncture. Yet, even this basic requirement of completing three tests was often not fulfilled because of the lack of sufficient funds for the author and the financial burden this would entail for the patients who had volunteered for free research treatment.

Before the results of our study were revealed in early 1972, there was no way of objectively evaluating the effectiveness of acupuncture for location technique as well as for time factors involved in the application of acupuncture in a manner scientifically acceptable to the Western-trained scientists. However, the results of our research indicate that there previously existed two opposing views,[3-8,10-67] that acupuncture causes vaso-dilation and that it causes vaso-constriction. These have now been clarified through our clinical research on human subjects. All of our research work on vascular response was carried out non-invasively before, during and after acupuncture. Specifically, our research indicates that a majority of the responses can be classified into three consecutive phases, i.e., the first of which is vaso-constriction, the second phase, quasi-control, and the third phase, vaso-dilation.[19,24-75,77]

Most of our results indicate that the beneficial effects of acupuncture are almost always associated with a significant generalized vaso-dilation of the capillaries and arterioles. For the first time, the mechanism by which high blood pressure is lowered has been clearly explained using the simple and accurate non-invasive technique of studying peripheral circulation as well as the brain circulation on the part of the forehead at which the blood supply comes mainly from the supra-orbital artery, the branch of the ophthalmic artery in the brain. Also, we have demonstrated in the laboratory that the generalized vaso-dilation of capillaries and arterioles induces significant decreases in serum concentration of triglycerides, phospholipids, and pre-B-lipids, and pre-B-lipoprotein, and less significant decreases in cholesterol and B-lipoprotein; these changes were particularly significant in those who had abnormally increased serum concentrations of lipid levels. Thus, it is now possible to evaluate the effectiveness of acupuncture and its techniques by the degree of induced generalized vaso-dilation and blood chemistry and CBC changes in the majority of cases, thereby eliminating the need to rely on subjective techniques for evaluation.

The author was able to demonstrate in the human being, for the first time non-invasively, acupuncture given in certain parts of the extremities in a branch of the internal carotid artery in the brain. Based on this information the author extended the research to treatment of patients with organic or transitional impairments of the brain circulation, such as in cases of migraine headaches, post-stroke patients, and patients whose circulation at the base of the eyeground is impaired, in those with nerve deafness, as well as psychiatric patients with symptoms of either severe anxiety or depression. In many of these cases, effectively given acupuncture induced significant improvement in the micro-circulation of the brain with significant change in blood chemistries with or without substantial improvement in the symptoms of the patients.

Much of the literature, both old and new, in Japanese and Chinese, describes the effectiveness of acupuncture in treating colds and some mild infectious diseases many of which appear to include various viral infections. A number of responsible professors in medical schools in the U.S., without having conducted any serious study in these matters, have discredited a lot of the claims associated with acupuncture as irresponsible and without scientific basis. These claims for the treatment of infectious diseases are rather non-specific, and there is a possibility that "Interferon" production by cells in the presence of certain viral infections might be increased by acupuncture. This possibility cannot be excluded until definite study is carried out to prove or disprove such speculation. On the other hand, the author observed a very slow but definite increase in the serum concentration of the gamma-globulin (more often in those who had colds or infections) which is indicative of the influence in the immune mechanism, particularly enhanced production of specific antibodies to specific viral or bacterial antigen. Again, this requires a lot of controlled study as well.

Judging from the author's research experience with acupuncture it becomes almost impossible to support or disregard each of the many claims of the beneficial effects of acupuncture without carrying out intensive research. However, acupuncture is not a panacea; it must be remembered that it has many limitations and, if not properly administered, can result in undesirable side-effects. For example, electro-acupuncture used without proper knowledge of its instruments and an understanding of the patho-physiology of the electro-acupuncture itself can produce vaso-constriction or necrosis of the body tissue surrounding the electrode and even breakage of the positive metal electrode within the body; in fact, we have begun to hear of such instances in the United States. Certainly then, minimum requirements for the design and use of the instruments and guidelines for precautions must be standardized to prevent unnecessary damage to the patients. At least, any electric stimulator sold for the purpose of electro-acupuncture, whether for use on an animal or a human, should indicate the typical wave pattern, polarity, pulse duration, amplitudes of both the plus and minus parts of the wave form, and the range of output impedance. If it is to be used with a part of surface electrodes without penetration of the skin, then the additional information of range of electrodes impedance should be indicated.

The purpose of the author's research was not simply to produce the beneficial effects of acupuncture but to explain the causes for the success as well as failure of acupuncture in producing such beneficial effects. The author found that acupuncture does not work in certain cases, and it is believed that the explanation for the success of acupuncture is necessarily linked to the explanation for its failure. Therefore, every study performed by the author, regardless of whether acupuncture produced beneficial effects, provided equally valuable information in formulating the author's theories on the mechanisms by which acupuncture works. In addition to the study of the mechanisms of pain and associated phenomena, the author's major research effort was devoted to the evaluation of the author's following hypotheses:

1) *Circulatory and Nervous Systems' Multi-Parameter Chemo-Humor-Neural Interaction Theory*, in which the author speculates

that the mechanical irritation of the cell membranes by acupuncture manipulation will increase the permeability of the cell membranes surrounding the acupunctured area and release certain chemical substances including enzymes from the interior to the exterior of the cells. This will first influence the acupunctured area, and then enter the circulatory system and affect distal parts of the body, including brain micro-circulation and lung circulation. Among such chemical substances,[55,67] some of the prostaglandins are most likely to be involved. Which kind of prostaglandin is released depends upon the part of the body to which acupuncture is administered. On the other hand, with histamine theory, it is impossible to explain why acupuncture improves bronchial asthma or histamine positive migraine headache.

a) A corollary to the theory is: *The greater the number of cells that are mechanically stimulated, the greater the amount of chemical substances that will be released, resulting in an enhanced acupuncture effect*—which was indirectly supported by the new criteria of evaluating the effectiveness of acupuncture through the author's research in measuring the degree of vaso-dilation in capillaries and arterioles.

b) *Mechanical stimulation is not limited to irritation with a needle,* but can also be produced by muscle contraction created by electrical excitation, or by pressure or squeezing effectively applied with one's finger. After application of one or more of these stimuli, effects similar to those of acupuncture should be expected. The author believes that this is most likely the basis for the effects of the Japanese *"Shiatsu."*

2) Introduction of the realistic broad concept of the Anatomical Functional Unit of "Neuro-Musculo-Vascular Unit" or "Vasculo-Neuro-Muscular Unit" rather than the widely used narrow concept of the "Neuro-Muscular Unit" is proposed to explain the mechanism of the relief of pain and relaxation of spastic muscles following the improvement of circulation by acupuncture. Most of the so-called musculo-skeletal pains are often associated with vascular disturbances which in turn irritate nerve fibers and create electrical excitation of both the sensory and motor nerve fibers. Excitation of some of the sensory nerve fibers is responsible for the pain sensation, while excitation of the motor nerve fibers induces contraction or spasm of the muscle fibers innervated by the particular nerve. This

contraction of muscles can be detected externally through palpation which reveals induration with tenderness. Such contraction further impairs the circulation by constricting the blood vessels, and the author believes, therefore, that relief of pain can be explained in some cases by considering the more practical concept of the functional "Neuro-Musculo-Vascular Unit" or "Vasculo-Neuro-Muscular Unit," which entails breaking the vicious pain cycle by improving the micro-circulation through acupuncture. Impairment of any one or more than one of these three interdependent factors can impair all three factors, resulting in various degrees of the "Vasculo-Neuro-Muscular Unit" dysfunction syndrome. The author has obtained the following supporting evidence in many patients who have arm pain shooting from the shoulder to the hand: After disappearance of the pain following acupuncture, if a blood pressure cuff is applied and pressure is raised beyond the systolic blood pressure level in the upper arm, the previously eliminated pain reappears within a few seconds after the occlusion of the artery by external pressure, but only in the part of the arm below the occluded area.

Our study on the effects of acupuncture on the nervous system showed that the effect on the threshold stimulation for pain sensation is often increased markedly, by a few hundred percent, most significantly in the acupunctured area but also, in some cases, in certain distal areas of the body. However, our results also show that there is only a slight decrease in conduction velocity of both the motor and sensory nerve fibers; this is usually not significant and is limited to the parts of the nerve fibers in very close proximity to the acupunctured location; the remaining parts of the same nerve fibers outside of the affected areas are not influenced by acupuncture. The well-known beneficial effects of acupuncture, such as pain relief or relaxation of a spastic muscle, will not appear until significant generalized vaso-dilation develops, usually within 30 seconds to a few minutes (although in some cases it occurs within 10 seconds) from the time of penetration of the skin. Therefore, considering the conduction velocity of the nerve fibers, the time required for the full development of the beneficial effects is quite difficult to explain in terms of the effects of acupuncture on the nervous system alone. Some people, based upon their general clinical impressions only, erroneously believe that the effects of acupuncture appear much more quickly than they actually do; even the simplest procedure of one needling requires at least 30 seconds from the time of insertion to the time of removal of the needle.

There are several entirely different theories about mechanisms in the genesis of pain,[39,54-65-67-74] including that of the well-publicized "gate control theory" of Melzack and Wall and its modified theory, "multi-gate control theory." However, none of these theories can explain all of the known clinical findings, and they lack direct experimental proof. As for pain relief mechanisms, in early 1972 the author proposed the following hypotheses:

1) Most pains are due to impairment of one or more of the parameters of the functional "Neuro-Musculo-Vascular Unit" or the "Vasculo-Neuro-Muscular Unit" (the term used depends upon which parameter receives the greatest emphasis). As we previously described, the improvement in circulation often breaks the vicious pain-maintenance cycle.

2) Excitation of the nerve fiber and its propagation for the transmission of the pain sensation can be inhibited artificially either by hyperpolarizing the transmembrane action potential and maintaining the hyperpolarized state, or by keeping the transmembrane action potential in its absolute or relative refractory periods. Some of this can be accomplished externally by applying electrical stimulation with high frequencies or a rapidly changing electro-magnetic field or capacitive current without direct contact between the electrode and body tissue. On the other hand, acupuncture effects can be obtained by a reduced rate of stimulation, as previously reported by the author in 1972.[40-41]

For the management of intractable pain, long-time study of the surgical procedure has not been too successful, particularly when it involves surgical severing in the various parts of the pathways of the nerve impulse for pain sensation between the peripheral nerve and the cerebral cortex. When the operation involves cutting a part of the spinal cord, the patient often develops loss of temperature and touch sensation. As a result, after the operation many patients suffer from unnecessary iatrogenic disabilities, even though they may have partial or complete relief from intractable pain. The worst problem is that in some cases the pain may come back a few years after the operation. Even with the simple laminectomy operation, there are many patients on whom the operation fails to eliminate intractable back pain with or without sciatic neuralgia syndrome. For instance, the author has had personal experience with a number of patients who had one or two laminectomy operations that failed to produce any improvement in back pain; but with acupuncture, relief of pain was induced almost immediately after the completion of a few minutes of continuous twirling of the needle in the area of tenderness or the pain trigger point. The author considers it important that before using any drastic surgical operation, for the sake of the patient, acupuncture should be considered as at least one possible choice of treatment and should at least be tried before proceeding with surgery. This is particularly important when the surgery involves risk of failure in eliminating pain and additional undesirable side-effects.

Even if acupuncture does not produce relief of pain, dorsal column stimulation, if properly performed, is still a better choice of treatment than drastic severing of the nerve pathway, since dorsal column stimulation has been shown to have an average success rate of about 65 percent. Thus about 35 percent of patients will end up without any relief of pain at all after the surgical implantation of the dorsal column stimulator and its electrodes. However, without going through the process of implanting the dorsal column stimulator, the effectiveness of dorsal column stimulation for managing intractable pain can be evaluated by electro-acupuncture using various frequencies of appropriate electrical impulses. Once electro-acupuncture is found to be effective in reducing or eliminating intractable pain during the application of impulses (with or without relief of pain following the discontinuation of the impulses), in those patients who do not desire implantation of the electrodes, effects similar to those of dorsal column stimulation can be obtained non-traumatically, without even sticking a needle in the body, with electric impulses through a pair of electro-conducting rubber electrodes placed on the body in the areas where electro-acupuncture was found to be effective.

Parts of the results of the author's research presented here give indirect supporting evidence for the author's hypotheses, and it is concluded that if the circulatory system as well as nervous system (although it is not an absolutely necessary condition) in the area is not drastically severed, acupuncture can be used for the treatment of some diseases and symptoms produced directly or indirectly by circulatory disturbances, particularly when other means of treatment have failed. However, much research remains to be done.

AUTHOR'S NOTE

Major parts of this article describing the original research of the author were presented at the University of Helsinki, University of Copenhagen, Upsala University, Karolinska Institute, University of Paris VI (formerly known as the Sorbonne), University of Poitiers, Heidelberg University, University of Geneva, etc., in 1972; at many medical schools and institutes (including Columbia University, Albert Einstein College of Medicine, New York University, University of Illinois, University of Texas, Emory University, University of Washington, etc.); at the First World Symposium on acupuncture and Chinese medicine in the United States; at International Congresses in Monte Carlo, Seoul, Korea, and at Hokkaida University; and at the anesthesiology meeting in Osaka, Japan, in 1973. This research has been supported by grants from the Heart Disease Research Foundation since 1971. The original manuscript of this chapter was submitted in December, 1972, and was revised in August, 1973. The following references were updated just before the final printing of this manuscript for the convenience of the readers.

REFERENCES

1. Tamba, Y. *Most Important Medical Methods* (*I-Shin-Ho*, written in Japanese with Chinese characters, 30 vols.), Japan, 982.
2. Hongo, M. *Important Useful Notes on Acupuncture and Moxibustion* (*Shin-Kyu Chou-Hou-Ki*, written in Japanese), Japan, 1718.
3. Manaka, Y., and Schmidt, Herbert. "Introductory Lecture on Acupuncture Methods for Physicians" ("I-Ka No Tame No Shin-Jutsu Nyu-Mon Kou-Za," written in Japanese), I-Do-No-Nihon-Sha, Oppama, Yokosuka, Japan, 1954.
4. Acupuncture-Moxibustion Outline Editorial Committee. *Outline of Chinese Acupuncture-Moxibustion Study* (*Chung Kuo Chen Chiu Hsiao Gai Yao*, written in Chinese), People's Health Publisher, Peking, 1964.
5. Shirota, B. *Practice of Acupuncture and Moxibustion Treatment with Main Emphasis on Clinical Cases* (*Chi-Ken-Rei O Shuto Shita Kyo Chi-Ryo-No Zitsusai*, written in Japanese, 2 vols.), Sou-Gen-Sha, Osaka, Japan, 1966.
6. Hyoudo, M. *New Methods of Treatment of Pain—Modern Application of Oriental Medicine* (*Itami No Atarashii Chiryohou' Toyou-Igaku No Kindaiteki Ouyou*, written in Japanese), Chugai-Igaku-Sha, Tokyo, 1969.

7. Kinoshita, H. *Sciatic Neuralgia and Acupuncture and Moxibustion* (*Zakatsu Shinkeitse To Shin-Kyo,* written in Japanese), Ido-no-Nihan-sha, Appama, Yokosuka, Japan, 1969.
8. Chu, L. *Study of New Acupuncture Moxibustion* (*Hsin Chen Chiu Hsiao,* written in Chinese), Shai Hua Wen Hua Fu Wu She, Hong Kong, 1970.
9. Manaka, Y. *Theory and Way of Thinking in Acupuncture-Moxibustion* (*Shin-Kyu No Ri-Ron To Kangae-Kata,* written in Japanese), Sou-Gen-Sha, Osaka, Japan, 1971.
10. Nagahama, Y.; Kinoshita, Hayeta; and Nakamura, Ryosuke. *New Research on Diagnosis and Treatments in Acupuncture and Moxibustion* (*Shin-Kyu Shin-Ryo No Shin-Kenkyu,* written in Japanese), Sou-Gen-Sha, Osaka, Japan, 1971.
11. Mann, F. *Acupuncture, The Ancient Chinese Art of Healing,* William Neinemann Medical Books, Ltd., London, 1971.
12. Omura, Y. "Patho-Physiology of Acupuncture Treatment, Part I," *The Acupuncture News Digest* (Original Research Section), National Acupuncture Research Society, vol. 3, no. 10, pp. 7-10, Oct. 1973. (Part 2, Ibid; vol. 3, no. 11. pp. 6-8, Nov. 1973.)
13. Omura, Y. *Acupuncture Medicine,* Japan Publications, Inc., Tokyo, Japan (In press).
14. Omura, Y. "Patho-Physiology of Acupuncture Treatment," *Critical Reviews in Clinical Laboratory Sciences,* Chemical Rubber Publishing Co., Cleveland, Ohio (In press).
15. Omura, Y. *Handbook of Acupuncture,* Chemical Rubber Publishing Co., Cleveland, Ohio (In press).
16. Shanghai Chinese Medicine Literature Research Institute (etd). *The Selected Essentials of Pulse Diagnosis* (*Mai Shew Yuan Yao,* written in Chinese), Business Publishing House (Shang Wu Yin Guan), Hong Kong, 1970.
17. Ren Ying Giu. *Chinese Medicine Pulsology—10 lectures* (*Chung I Mai Xue Shi Jiang,* written in Chinese) Ta-Ping Shu-Ju, Hong Kong, 1970.
18. Yamanobe, N. *Guide for the Pulse Diagnosis Method* (*Miyaku-Hou Tebiki Sou,* written in Japanese), Tokyo, Japan, 1771.
19. Omura, Y., and Lee, K. "Applications of Ultra-Miniature Photoelectric Plethysmographic Sensors with a Very Short Response Time to the Non-Traumatic Study of the Circulatory System," *Transactions of the American Society for Artificial Internal Organs* 17:392-404, 1971.
20. Omura, Y., and Lee, K. "Non-Traumatic Study of Cardio-Vascular (VC) Systems Under Various Clinical Conditions wth Ultra-Miniature Reflection Type Photoelectric Plethysmographic Sensors," *Abstracts,* vol. 1, of the 18th annual meeting of the American Society for Artificial Internal Organs, p. 37, April, 1972.
21. Omura, Y. "Invasive and Non-Invasive Studies of the Effects of Drugs," *Abstract* of the 5th International Congress of Pharmacology,

1972, (and 17-page news release of the paper prepared at the request of the Congress, held at San Francisco, April, 1972).
22. Omura, Y. "Effects of Acupuncture on the Cardio-Vascular System," studies on Essential Hypertension and Blood Chemistry; Abstracts of the 3rd World Congress of Acupuncture, held at Seoul, Korea, pp. 208-209, September, 1973.
23. Omura, Y., and Lee, K. "The Effects of Acupuncture (AC) on Cardio-Vascular and Nervous Systems," *Abstracts*, vol. 2, of the 19th annual meeting of the American Society for Artificial Internal Organs, p. 48, April, 1973.
24. Omura, Y. "Effects of Acupuncture on Blood Pressure, Leukocytes and Serum Lipids and Lipoproteins in Essential Hypertension," presented on April 11, 1974, and Abstract published in the Federation Proceedings for Experimental Biology, p. 430, March, 1974.
25. Akabane, K. *Method of Hinaishin* (written in both Japanese and English), Ido-No-Nihppon-Sha, Oppama, Yokosuka, Japan, 1964.
26. Nakatani, Y. *General Theory of Ryo-Do-Raku*, Ryo-Do-Raku Research Institute, Japan, 1966.
27. Travell, J., and Bobb, A.L. "Mechanism of Relief of Pain in Sprains by Local Injection Techniques," Federation proceedings, vol. 6, p. 378, March, 1947.
28. Travell, J. "Basis for the Multiple Uses of Local Block of Somatic Trigger Areas (Procaine Infiltration and Ethyl Chloride Spray)," *Mississippi Medical Journal* 71:13-21, 1949.
29. Travell, J., and Rinzler, S.H. "The Myofacial Genesis of Pain," *Post-Graduate Medicine*, vol. 11, no. 5, pp. 425-434, 1952.
30. Bonica, J. *Management of Pain*, Lea and Febiger, Philadelphia, 1953.
31. Sola, A. F., and William, R.L. "Myofacial Pain Syndromes," *Neurology*, vol. 6, no. 2, pp. 91-95, Feb., 1966.
32. Animal Research Institute of the Chinese Science Institute. "Method of Auricular Acupuncture Treatment" ("Er-Chen-Liao-Fa," written in Chinese), Shang Wu Yin Shu Kuan, Hong Kong, 1972.
33. Nogier, P.F.M. *Treatise of Auriculotherapy*, Maison-neuve S.A. Moulins-les-metz, France, 1972.
34. Mori, H. *Immediately Clinically Useful Acupuncture Introduction* (*Rin-Shiyo Ni Gugu Yaku-datsu Hari Niu-mon*, written in Japanese), Ido-No-Nihon-Shu, Oppama, Yokosuka, Japan, 1973.
35. Yanagiya, D. *Illustrated Explanation of Practical Techniques in Acupuncture and Moxibustion* (*Zu Setsu Shin Kiyu Kitsugi*, written in Japanese), Ido-No-Nihon-Hsa, Oppama, Yokosuka, Japan, 1948.
36. Wu Hui Ping. *Acupuncture Moxibustion Medicine* (*Chen Chiu I Hsueh*), Hsin-Ya-Chu-Ban-She, Taihoku, Taiwan, 1968.
37. Feng, T.Y. *Study of Electro-Acupuncture and Moxibustion Treatments* (*Tien Chen Chiu Chih Liao Hsiao*, written in Chinese), Shang Wu Ying Shu Kuan, Hong Kong, 1970.
38. Acupuncture Anesthesia Editorial Committee. *Acupuncture Anes-*

thesia (Analgesia) (*Zhen Ci Ma Aui,* written in Chinese), Shanghai People's Publisher, Shanghai, 1972.
39. Weddell, A.G.M. "Activity pattern hypothesis for sensation of pain," in R.G. Crenell (ed.), *Neural Physiopathology, Some Relationships of Normal to Altered Nervous System Activity.* A Hoeber Medical Book, Harper & Row, pp. 134-177, 1962.
40. Noordenbos, W. *Pain.* Amsterdam: Elsevier, 1959.
41. Melzack, R., and Wall, P.D. "Pain Mechanisms: A New Theory," *Science* 150:971-979, 1965.
42. Melzack, R. *The Puzzle of Pain.* Basic Books Publishing Co., New York, 1973.
43. Li, Choh-luh."Neurological basis of pain and its possible relationship to acupuncture analgesia," *American Journal of Chinese Medicine* 1, no. 1, pp. 61-72, January, 1973.
44. Sweet, William H., and Wepsic, James G. "Treatment of chronic pain by stimulation of fibers of primary afferent neuron," Trans. American Neurological Assoc. 93:103-7, 1968.
45. Shealy, C. Norman; Mortimer, J. Thomas; and Hagforst, Norman R. "Dorsal column electroanalgesia," *Journal of Neurosurgery* 32:560-564, May, 1970.
46. Wall, Patrick D., and Wall, William H. "Temporary abolition of pain in man," *Science,* pp. 108-09, 1967.
47. Sawe, Urbain. "Pain in acute myocardial infraction: a study of 137 patients in a coronary care unit," *Acta med. scand.* 190:79-81, 1971.
48. Shealy, C. Norman. "The physiological substrate of pain," *Headache,* pp. 101-08, October, 1966.
49. Collins, William F., and Randt, Clark T. "Midbrains evoked responses relating to peripheral unmyelinated or 'C' fibers in cat," *Journal of Neurophysiology* 23:47-53, January, 1960.
50. Smorto, Mario P., and Basmajian, John V. *Clinical Electroneurography,* Williams & Wilkin Co., Baltimore, 1972.
51. Casey, K.L., and Melzack, R. "Neural mechanisms of pain: a conceptual method," in *New Concepts in Pain and Its Clinical Management,* E. Leong Way (ed.), F. A. Davis Co., Philadelphia, 1967, pp. 13-31.
52. Lim, R.K.S. "Pharmacologic viewpoint of pain and analgesia," in *New Concepts in Pain and Its Clinical Management,* E. Leong Way (ed.), F.A. Davis Co., Philadelphia, 1967, pp. 33-47.
53. Bonica, John J. "Management of intractable pain," in *New Concepts in Pain and Its Clinical Management,* E. Leong Way (ed.), F.A. Davis Co., Philadelphia, 1967, pp. 155-167.
54. Sweet, William H. "Neurosurgical management of pain," in *New Concepts in Pain and Its Clinical Management,* E. Leong Way (ed.), F.A. Davis Co., Philadelphia, 1967, pp. 169-185.
55. Rocha e Silva, M., and Garcia Leme, Jr. *Chemical Mediators of the Acute Inflammatory Reaction,* Pergamon Press, New York, 1972.

56. Joffey, J.J. "The present status of the lymphocyte problem," *Lancet I*, pp. 206-211, 1962.
57. Lewis, T., and Grant, R.T. "Vascular reactions of the skin to injury, II. The liberation of a histamine-like substance in injured skin: the underlying cause of factitious urticaria and of wheels produced by burning, and observations upon the nervous control of certain skin reactions," *Heart* 11:119-209, 1923-24.
58. Lewis, T. *The Blood Vessels of the Human Skin and their Responses*, Shaw & Sons, Ltd., London, 1927.
59. Hilton, S.M. "A peripheral arterial conducting mechanism underlying dilation of the femoral artery and concerned in functional vasodilation in skeletal muscle," *J. Physiol.* 149:93-111, London, 1959.
60. Hilton, S.M. "Experiments on the post-contraction hyperaemia of skeletal muscle," *J. Physiol.* 102:230-45, London, 1953.
61. Galton, D.J. *The Human Adipose Cell (A Model for Errors in Metabolic Regulation)*, Appleton-Century Crofts, New York, 1971.
62. Feldberg, W., and Lewis, G.P. "The action of peptides on the adrenal medulla. Release of adrenaline by bradykinin and angiotessin," *J. Physiol.* 171:98-108, London, 1964.
63. Anderson, G.G., and Speroff, L. "Prostaglandins," *Science* 171: 502-504, 1971.
64. Chen, J.Y.P. "Acupuncture," pp. 65-90, and "Pharmacology," pp. 91-106, as two sections of "Chapter 1, Chinese Medicine Through the Ages" in *Medicine and Public Health in the People's Republic of China*, J.R. Quinn (ed.), DHEW Publication No. (NIH) 72-67, N.I.H. Bethesda, Maryland, 1972.
65. Nertermans, S.L.H. "Measurement of the pain threshold determined by electrical stimulation and its clinical application—part 1, Method and factors possibly influencing the pain threshold," *Neurology* 14: 1071-85, 1971.
66. Remwell, P., and Shaw, J.E. "Prostaglandins," *Annals of the New York Academy of Sciences*, vol. 180 (more than 50 articles by many authors), New York, 1971.
67. Serizawa, K. *Science of Acupuncture and Moxibustion* (*Shin-Kyu No Kagaku*, written in Japanese), Ishiyaku Publishing Co., Tokyo, Japan, 1959.
68. *Mainichi Life*, Staff writer (ed). Special Issue on Everything on the Shiatsu Treatment (Tokushu, Shiatsu Ryoho No Subete, written in Japanese), March, 1972.
69. *Mainichi Life*, Special Issue, Part 2: Present Day Acupuncture Moxibustion, several authors, May, 1972.
70. Spiegel, Herbert. "An Eye-Roll Test for Hypnotizability," *American Journal of Clinical Hypnosis* 15, no. 1, (July, 1972), pp. 25-28.
71. Wageneder, F.M., St. Schuy, (ed.). *Electrotherapeutic Sleep and Electroanesthesia*, vol. 2, Excerpta Medica, Amsterdam, 1970.

72. Omura, Y.; Lee, K.; and Jeronimo, M. "Stimulation of excitable cell membrances by capacitive current and rapidly-changing electro-magnetic field without direct contact between electrodes and the cells," *Federation Proceedings* 31, no. 2, presented at the annual scientific meeting of the FASEB at Atlantic City on April 14, 1972.
73. Omura, Y. "The relationship between the transmembrane action potential and the voltage-time-dependent negative resistance characteristics of the voltage-current curves of excitable pacemaker and nonpacemaker cell membranes," *Transactions of the New York Academy of Sciences,* Series II, vol. 33, no. 5,pp. 467-518 and Appendix i-xiv, May, 1971.
74. Omura, Y. "Effects of acupuncture on the nervous system: studies on the threshold stimulation and conduction velocities of motor and sensory nerve fibers" in Abstracts of the 3rd World Congress of Acupuncture, held at Seoul, Korea, pp. 209-210, Sept., 1973.
75. Omura, Y. "Cardiovascular responses to acupuncture," one-hour talk presented as the guest speaker of the research section of the First World Symposium on Acupuncture and Chinese Medicine held in San Francisco, on Sept. 14, 1974; abstract published in the Proceedings of the First World Symposium on Acupuncture and Chinese Medicine in *American Journal of Chinese Medicine* 2, no. 1, pp. 112-113, 1974.
76. Peng, A.T.C.; Omura, Y.; Cheng, H.C.; and Blancato, L.S. "Acupuncture for relief of chronic pain and surgical analgesia," *The American Surgeon* 40, no. 1, pp. 50-53, January, 1974.
77. Omura, Y. "Clinical applications and limitations of acupuncture (with special emphasis on the management of pain) and its patho-physiological basis and effects of acupuncture on the cardiovascular and nervous systems" in *Management of Pain,* J. Bonica (ed.), Lea & Febiger, Philadelphia, (in press).

CHAPTER VII

ACUPUNCTURE AND PAIN

In 1967 Dr. Hans Noterman of the Netherlands developed an electrical system for measuring pain, based on electrical discharge in the brain following the application of painful stimuli; and in 1968 Shealy and co-workers developed a concept of PSAD, the prolonged small fiber after discharge, which gives us a little more substantial basis for pain measurement. But even these advanced methods did not eliminate the variables, since they were either effective only in cats or relied on human subjects to interpret what was felt.

Because of these variables, an accurate objective system is mandatory. Many factors influence the entity called pain; *Science* magazine describes pain not as a sensation but as a "modality class which is a linguistic label for a rich variety of experiences and responses."

The common factors which affect pain are conditioning, emotion, memory; attention, distraction, religion, politics, and other convictions (immolation); fear, fatigue, physical status, psychiatric status (as in masochism, where pain is even enjoyed). There are some pain states that defy explanation, such as phantom limb and causalgia.

As a result of this complexity, treatment methods have ranged from analgesia, narcotics, and surgery, to conditioning, psychotherapy, hypnotism, religion, quackery, and witchcraft. Too often all have failed. One motor vehicle accident left the patient with a severely painful shoulder. In succession, he underwent the following operations without relief: amputation, neurectomy, rhizotomy, cordotomy, lobotomy, thalamotomy, and finally ECT. Although this is an extreme example, many other recorded cases reflect this type of failure.

"The nature of pain has been the subject of bitter controversy since the turn of the century," says a prominent scientific writer in the beginning of his paper, and he immediately proposes another new theory that is now controversial. Nowadays neurologists quickly dismiss the specificity theory which holds that pain is a specific, like touch or temperature, or that it has its own system of transmission from the receptor to the brain.

The pattern theory is another theory which modernists dispute. It claims that non-specific receptors carrying the impulse by non-specific fibers cause the formation of a pattern of nerve transmission which the brain interprets as pain.

Both theories have been found deficient in explaining some of the phenomena of pain such as summation, time delay, phantom limb pain, and other causalgias. And, as previously mentioned, if the physiologic model of the nervous system that we all more or less accept were to hold, how do we explain the persistence of pain when as much as the entire anatomical pain-causing system has been removed surgically?

So much for pain theories. What about acupuncture? The Chinese theorists, inscrutable as ever, also had a wonderful time explaining the unexplainable. First there is the meridian theory.

This is also usually referred to as the *chinglo* theory and is the standard basis for classical Chinese acupuncture, dating back two to five thousand years. It postulates that on the body there are hundreds of points, connected by paired bilateral imaginary lines called meridians, of which there are 12 paired and 2 unpaired. It asserts that a life force, *chi* or *ki*, circulates through these meridians once every 24 hours, starting with the lungs and going through the other organs via their meridians. It states that illness in the organs is caused by too much or too little *ki*, and the needling can restore the balance between the *ki*-deficient organs and the *ki*-excess organs, and thus restore health. It lists combinations, almost recipes, for using different spots in different diseases, and has a variety of times, places, suns, moons, and other instructions regarding the administration of these needles.

As we have stated, this theory is a remarkably attractive system of antique mythology, laced with poetry and tradition. But it is not science.

Neither is Professor Kim Bong Han's theory, which is based on a similar foundation of fantasy, and which to date no one, not even with an electron microscope, has been able to verify.

Professor Kim Bong Han, of North Korea, has stated that there is a fourth circulation, other than nerves, arteries, veins, and lymphatics, which is composed of channels containing a colorless fluid rich in colloids. These Bonghans tubules, as they are called, connect the acupuncture points and are the meridians discussed in Chinese literature. In addition, surrounding most organs, and filling the acupuncture points, are cells which seem to be specialized for conductivity and which are again modestly called Bonghans cells; the peripheral Bonghans cells and the deeper organ cells are connected by communicating tubules, thus giving a complete circulation, and accounting for the remotely connected cause and effect seen in acupuncture phenomena. Staining these cells and injecting them with radioisotopes are two of the "scientific" bases for accepting this theory.

The French and the Italian acupuncturists likewise subscribe to the meridian theory, and both schools have developed punctascopes or tobiscopes which identify points in the skin of generally loose consistency, high electrical resistance, and unique spectroscopic qualities.

In a review of other theories, Toyama and Nishizawa contend that the acupuncture points correspond quite closely to the "trigger zones" of Sir Henry Head. According to Head's postulate, cutaneous pain felt in visceral disease is due to the anatomical fact of the afferent pain fibers and the spinal nerves entering the spinal cord at the same segment or dermatome. Here it is presupposed an interchange takes place at the internuncial junction.

Moss of England agrees with this view and says most of these points are between the buttocks and the scapula, thus perpetuating the idea of points in the skin.

Mandell of the U.S. notes that stimulation of the amygdala produced an excess of 17 hydroxycortocoid release. If we couple the findings of Kassil with the reports of Mandell we arrive at a hormone theory of acupuncture where it is thought that the effect of acupuncture is due to the cerebrum stimulated by the needling, in turn stimulating the thalamus, hypothalamus, and limbic system. ACTH, to the equivalent of 25 international units, can be produced, assert Boeva and his associates, through the reticular activating system, if what he calls "stimulation acupuncture" is used. The amygdala, stimulated by a stimulated cerebrum, can also produce an excess of 17 hydroxycortocoid release, while the limbic system can generate other impulses to the hypothalamus and affect the entire endocrine system subordinate to the anterior pituitary. Boeva feels that stimulation by different needle points on the skin generates impulses which travel through the somato-visceral neuronal synapses in the spinal cord and on to the viscera. Selective stimulation of dominant components of the visceral nerves, either sympathetic or parasympathetic, influences and adjusts the function of the autonomic neurons system and produces body changes.

The evidence to support this theory stems from Russia, namely the work of Dr. Grashchenko, who demonstrated that acupuncture could affect the blood content of asthmatics and peptic ulcer patients by lowering to normal the values of acetylcholine, acetylcholinesterase, diamine oxidase, epinephrine and norepinephrine.

Another Russian theory is the reflex theory, which was presented by Kassil and associates at the Reflex Therapy Laboratory in Moscow. Each area of the skin surface has a representative area in the cerebral cortex. Stimulation of various kinds, such as by acupuncture or moxibustion, on specific skin localities, acts on its representative area in the cortex, after traveling there through specific pathways. That it alters cerebral cortical function is obvious, since it is shown to produce changes in the electroencephalogram. Dr. Henri Jarricot, of France, supports this with his "Reflexotherapy."

Well, what about all these theories? A new one comes out every minute. Dr. Jack Geiger, visiting China, brought out another one wherein he states that it's the neuromuscular end-plates that are crucial. Dr. Melzack, in his new book, *The Puzzle of Pain*, talks of other things—hyperstimulation, analgesia, and a central biasing mechanism.

The author's lecture below, excerpted from a University of Wisconsin symposium on acupuncture, might clarify some additional points. The date is November 19, 1974:

Acupuncture, Hypnosis and Pain

The pain controversy has been raging in this country and abroad for more than fifty years, and, at this point, we still have no real definition of what pain is. We also have no real definition of what hypnosis is and lack a positive methodology of acupuncture. Some attempts have been made to explain these interrelated subjects, for none of which we have a single definition, from scattered experimental work—some good, some bad.

Obviously, in most areas we have no "hard facts" concerning acupuncture because they are virtually impossible to achieve in the absence of final facts about both hypnosis and pain, the basic substrata for the acupuncture effects. It is somewhat of a presumption to expect to produce these hard facts in acupuncture on the basis of only a few years of effort. Therein lies the unfairness of some medical societies with which I have been in contact throughout the country whose criteria are rigidly bound to hard facts. However, I am slowly coming back to respect the attitude of the American Medical Association (in this case one of fairmindedness), which has exposed and published facts about acupuncture that are both positive and negative, at least presenting both sides for consideration by the medical community.

Medical school textbooks contain a diagram that shows the pathway of pain. There is also a pathway for temperature, a pathway for vibration, and paths of the various sensory functions. Almost all have been more or less neurologically traced out and verified. But the *pain* pathways have never been successfully delineated *in toto*, and have never been successfully demonstrated even with surgery. This is obvious from the clinical records of pain phenomena such as summation, reverberation, phantom limb and others. Conditions in this category cannot be explained from those very nice, neat, cut-and-dry anatomical and neurological diagrams we all studied.

The current definition of pain as expressed by Dr. Ronald Melzack of Montreal, perhaps the foremost researcher in pain in the Western world, is found in a book I highly recommend: *The Puzzle of Pain*. It is interesting that he would write an authoritative book on pain in 1974 and call it the "puzzle" of pain, not what pain is. In the past, Dr. Melzack contributed one-half of the Melzack-Wall "gate" theory which could have established the relationship of pain to acupuncture. Today neither Dr. Melzack nor Dr. Wall, for differing reasons, believes their gate theory any longer relates to acupuncture, postulating a "central biasing mechanism" and "hyperstimulation analgesia" as the important etiologic precepts.

In *The Puzzle of Pain,* Dr. Melzack says that pain does not travel along the specific tracts we had been taught in school. For example, in some cases pain has persisted even though the entire pain tract from sense organs to cerebrum was removed. First, the limb from where the pain was supposed to be issuing was removed, then a neurotomy, rhizotomy, cordotomy, even an extirpation of the nervous tissue right up the cerebrum, and finally electric-shock therapy were performed! But, according to the patient, the pain persisted. Several cases of this type have been reported, thus defying our neat neurological explanation of the pain pathway. Melzack indicates that, rather than one, there are really two ascending pathways and one descending pathway, and that even these pathways are not yet clearly and completely demarcated. The two ascending pathways are the sensory-discriminative (Neo-spinothalamic) and the motivational-affective (Reticular Formation); the one descending pathway is the cognitive-evaluative; in gross terms the ascending pathways are neurologic, whereas the descending pathway may be more psychic and may involve some biochemical as well as neurologic factors. The three pathways are further described by Dr. Melzack and give us a clear-cut demonstration that in this particular instance what we have accepted as hard facts all our medical lives are not really hard facts at all.

A re-reading of Pitken's book *Conduction Anesthesia* would astonish the reader who would note how many times the author says, "it is presumed that," and, "it is supposed that," and "current evidence leads us to believe." Perhaps, by overlooking such statements, we have forgotten that there is a great deal of presumptive evidence rather than hard facts in all our medical texts, particularly in the area of neurology. Obviously, we do not have access, except by indirect means, to human beings as experimental animals. Where, then, can we actually do the kind of research we want to do, particularly neurologic in nature? The answer is nowhere, and thus research has been dragging. Furthermore, translating our animal research into human research can be difficult and often misleading. And so with this severe impediment, we have really been unable to progress in pain definition, leaving it somewhat in limbo.

As to hypnosis: how much do we really know about hypnosis? I was a participant in the hypnosis controversy when it took place twenty years or more ago. A medical student at that time, I published one of the first articles on hypnosis admitted into a medical magazine. In Chicago, one of the investigators under whom I worked could not get the word *hypnosis* printed in the American Medical Association *Journal,* even in the form of an inclusion in the letters to the editor!

At that time, back in 1956, the hypnosis avant-garde was facing the identical problem we are facing now with acupuncture—namely, scientists and quasi-scientists demanding hard facts. Eventually some were produced, although it is difficult to say how concrete they really were.

Hypnosis today is established to the point where one can apply it in practice without being labeled a quack. This was not the case twenty-five years ago. And today, many of us are being labeled quacks if we talk about acupuncture. We are faced with the same antagonism on the part of the same people who insist on the same sort of thing they insisted on years ago. Surprisingly, a few hypnotists have added their voices to the opposition, despite the fact that we are years into hypnosis now and still don't have much solid data. We have statistics on success rates, we have defined a few parameters, but I think a great deal of the research could not be classified as hard fact.

Yet we all use hypnosis; we use it even when we don't think we're using it and even though advanced physiologists and others can't give us a clear-cut definition. There are theories, many theories, but really no hard facts. And yet, without being able to define hypnosis, some are ready to say that it is equivalent to acupuncture, which we also can't define, because of the similarity in certain areas of pain, for which we are still awaiting a definition. What a treadmill!

The hypnotic situation breaks down into three factors: aura, motivation, and probability of success. A patient's response to hypnosis depends on whether these three factors are in play; if strongly in play, a patient can be hypnotized. The patient does not have to be somnambulistically hypnotized, which is another consideration entirely. We are not involved here with the idea of Svengali and Trilby: a hypnotist waving his hand, whereupon the patient goes into a trance. A true hypnotic trance is possible to achieve only with a relatively small portion of the hypnotic population—fifteen percent at the maximum, and five percent at the minimum. The variability depends on the hypnotist, but it is generally agreed that not more than fifteen percent of the population can be made to go into a trance state by even the most successful hypnotist in the world.

Strangely enough, the vaudeville hypnotist knows these statistics. When performing his act, he gets a group of people on stage and does a simple hypnotic test, such as telling them to clasp their hands and then seeing which ones can't pull them apart at his suggestion that they cannot. By this method he identifies the somnambules. Out of about twenty people he can find perhaps two or three. He knows that is fairly close to the percentage that is somnambulistic, and he furthermore knows he can work best with them. But explain why? He leaves that to the scientists. If you find a subject who is a somnambule, you can do the most remarkable demonstrations and experiments; but where are the hard facts to explain the phenomenon?

A somnambule can be operated on without any chemical anesthetic at all. At the New York State Society of Anesthesiologists' meeting in 1958, a demonstration took place that may well have tipped the balance in favor of hypnosis in this country, for, coincidentally, it became approved shortly afterward. Dr. Vincent Collins, the Director of Anesthesiology at St. Vincent's Hospital, and I supervised four major operations. They were performed under hypnosis with an anesthetic, without any premedication and without any acupuncture. However, these four people were selected because they were somnambules; we knew that almost anything could be done with such individuals under hypnosis if the proper suggestions were made and the proper ritual performed.

Hypnotic surgery is an important technique, and there is no basis for a valid argument on acupuncture versus hypnosis. We know that we can use hypnosis successfully in surgery, but only in five to fifteen percent of all cases. Chinese statistics talk of eighty to ninety percent success with acupuncture, but realistically we might expect a sixty to seventy percent success in this country. Between this percentage and the fifteen percent of hypnosis, something important is happening. Some other mechanism of analgesia is undoubtedly at work.

Every doctor who maintains an office, seeing patients on a person-to-person basis (we exclude research patients), has been practicing hypnosis whether he knows it or not. Every therapeutic situation in medicine is a hypnotic situation, because it contains the three elements mentioned above: aura, motivation, and probability of success. Despite recent adverse publicity, polls show that physicians in this country are one of the mostly highly respected groups, if not *the* most highly respected group. That aura is working for the physician to help his therapy.

As for motivation, the patient who has come to see you voluntarily is indicating a great deal about his psychiatric profile: he has come to see the physician because he obviously wants to get well. If this patient were masochistic or determined to destroy himself, he would do what a great many people do. His internal dialogue might run this way: "I don't want to know what I have, maybe cancer. If I do, I don't want to know about it." This patient is psychiatrically motivated, but ordinarily the patient who comes to see a doctor in the average therapeutic situation is motivated towards getting well.

The third element, the probability of success, is fairly evident —the patient has come to you because he has heard of you through some friend or fellow physician, or he has heard of your capabilities through the medical media. The patient with stomach trouble will want to go to the stomach specialist. The probability-of-success factor is very high, because the patient has come to the person he considers most capable of helping him, and he already is partially hypnotized by his acceptance of this physician as the potential healer. Thus, these three factors in operation in the therapeutic situation add up to a hypnotic situation, whether it is so labelled or not.

What probably has done most harm to acupuncture in this country has been the term itself, associating it medically with inscrutable, mysterious, and sometimes spurious Eastern lore. We could call it quackupuncture, or even arguepuncture. Right now that may be the most valuable term. What most people are doing is arguing about it, and not from viewpoints that are totally devoted, dedicated or selfless, either. A great many of the physicians arguing against acupuncture are trying to protect a hypnosis practice, or a pain empire or a steroid practice. A good acupuncturist could clear out their offices in a few days.

Hypnosis patients would find that acupuncture has a much more prolonged effect and is a simpler method. Sometimes it seems to produce a parallel result, but it works by a different mechanism. Exactly what the mechanism is, is not known at this time, but it is not the neurophysiologic mechanism proposed by either Chinese or American workers, except perhaps in the area of pain. It is definitely not explained by the gate theory. Dr. Robert O. Becker, an orthopedic surgeon from Syracuse, New York, has this to say about a possible biologic mechanism of acupuncture:

> The therapeutic technique of acupuncture has no known basis in fact; neither the points nor meridians have any neuroanatomical relationship, and the simple insertion of a needle unaccompanied by any chemical agent appears to be of trivial significance. We reject the philosophical, vitalistic explanations of Yang and Yin, but have been unable to provide any adequate explanation based upon our current scientific knowledge. In this situation, logic dictates two conclusions: either acupuncture has no basis in biological fact, and its effects can be ascribed solely to suggestion; or it is real, but it acts via a heretofore undescribed physiological mechanism.
>
> For the past 15 years, our laboratory has been concerned with the factors that initiate and control healing mechanisms. During that time we have slowly accumulated evidence for the existence of such a previously unknown mechanism, until today we believe we can describe a complete control system functioning in concert with, but separate from, the nervous system. This has proven to be a powerful theoretical tool that is applicable to many poorly understood biological phenomena, including acupuncture.

I am associated in New York with the Postgraduate Center for Mental Health, an institution dedicated to mental care with an extremely large staff of psychiatrists and mental health professionals. Carrying a work load of approximately 1500 patient hours a week, it is a veritable department store of psychiatric opinion, and very strongly oriented toward hypnosis. The medical director is Dr. Lewis R. Wolberg, one of the foremost proponents of hypnosis in this country and the author of innumerable standard texts on the subject. I've had a difficult time convincing him of the efficiency of acupuncture, but finally some studies that I did won him over.

From January to May 1972, 132 cases were referred to me from upstairs at the PGMH. My office, in keeping with the status accorded acupuncture at that time, was in the basement. It was referred to as "down there"; pretty close to Lucifer, obviously. Anyway, down there was where they sent these poor patients. They sent me the flunk-outs from hypnosis programs and many flunk-outs from the psychoanalytic programs. Some of them had

had been on the couch so long they might have been referrals from the Great Sigmund himself. I saw the widest assortment of patients imaginable, all looking for relief in my office—what amounted to a medical last port-of-call.

I was floundering around myself, grasping for a few factual anchors. They were very scarce. Through the grapevine, I was receiving the *Peking Review* regularly. The *Peking Review* at that time was being published in Chinese; only recently has it started coming out in English as well. It can be described as a medical newspaper with the scientific flavor of *Medical World News.* It gives you capsules, but not the detailed information the scientific mind would look for: "Exactly how did you do it? Exactly what are the controls?" I was using it as my reference because that was all I could get.

There were some references on the treatment of mental disease by acupuncture as well as notes on acupuncture analgesia for surgery, and so I embarked on a program aimed at determining the relationship between hypnosis and acupuncture in the psychiatric area.

The Stanford Hypnotizability and the Harvard Hypnotizability tests were part of the work-up on each patient. These are not physical tests, like the eyeball tests, but, rather, written tests which can be purchased. Anyone intending to do acupuncture should include them in order to learn more about the patient's psychiatric profile and, possibly, which modality one is working with.

After these and other advance tests, I proceeded to treat the patients to the best of my ability, explaining very carefully to them that this was totally experimental, that we didn't know very much about it in this country, and that I doubted if they even knew that much more about it in China other than what thousands of years of empiric observation had taught them.

My results were spotty; as a well-known anesthesiologist observed, if you get good results you're a good observer, if you get bad results you're a bad acupuncturist. (This remark has been attributed to Dr. Ronald Katz, now Professor and Chairman of the Department of Anesthesiology at U.C.L.A.)

Among the 132 patients, I found only a casual relationship between the degree of hypnotizability and the success of my acupuncture. Totally random, it didn't relate to age, weight, height, sex, indoctrination (they all got the same indoctrination).

There were patients whom I could hypnotize very easily; my expectancy was that these patients would get good relief with acupuncture, but they didn't. There were other patients that I could not hypnotize who got good relief from acupuncture. Neither could an inverse relationship be established. It was totally random.

On the other hand, Spiegel and Katz, at Columbia University, in 112 patients found a high correlation between the degree of hypnotizability and positive acupuncture results. Furthermore, Choh-Lu Li at the N.I.H. found acupuncture to be less than effective in 14 patients. My opinion is that, except as a preliminary sample, we cannot draw firm conclusions from any of these studies. In mental health, you really need to accumulate data on thousands of patients before you can assess your results.

Are these hard facts? Are they preliminary samples that should be pursued in an attempt to find out this relationship? Is it, in fact, an important relationship? These questions are not academic when scientific journals are only too ready to label acupuncture as "hokum." We must not allow this practice unless it is finally and absolutely proven to have no inherent value for anyone anywhere. Too many permanent advances in medicine, hypnosis included, were first greeted with the "hokum" label, and we must take such lessons to heart. Hopefully, acceptance of acupuncture will follow the same route that enabled hypnosis to be recognized.

Excerpt from the *Salt Lake City, Utah, Tribune*, February 18, 1974:

> . . . Dr. Katz said acupuncture is a phenomenon that parallels hypnosis, but that he really doesn't know how it works.
>
> But, he added, some work done in the name of acupuncture is really hypnosis. "Instead of the ball and chain or watch you just watch the twirling needles," Dr. Katz said. However, he also emphasized that not all acupuncture can be ruled as hypnosis . . .

As of this writing, not only Dr. Katz now feels that there is a difference between acupuncture and hypnosis. Dr. Patrick Wall also has abandoned his earlier ideas that acupuncture is not anything but pure hypnosis. Dr. Melzack agrees that there is a mechanism there that is outside the hypnotic area, and only die-hard non-stickers who have "observed" the phenomenon of acupuncture remotely can maintain their original premise.

CHAPTER VIII

SOME PSYCHIATRIC AND HYPNOTIC CONSIDERATIONS OF ACUPUNCTURE

Lewis R. Wolberg

Dean, Postgraduate Center for Mental Health, New York

[*Reprinted from the* Proceedings of the First Acupuncture Workshop, *June 3, 1972, at the Postgraduate Center for Mental Health.*]

Concerning acupuncture, I am interested, excited, hopeful—as you are. But we must again sound the warning that an attitude of scientific skepticism is absolutely mandatory in evaluating any kind of new procedure. We often go overboard whenever a new instrumentality is introduced into the field. On the basis of our hope that a new modality will solve our problems, we are inclined to be overoptimistic about its value. This doesn't mean we have to stop experimenting. A good deal of controversy about acupuncture—what it is, how it works, its values—has invaded the field. Contradictory statements pro and con have appeared in the professional and popular press and over the air. I would like to address myself to some of these contradictory statements, especially those that relate to the hypnotic aspects of acupuncture.

How can we apply the tactics of scientific method to any procedure like acupuncture? First, we need an unprejudiced compilation of facts and information; second, we engage in the formulation of reasonable hypothesis; third, we strive for the retention of objectivity in observation; and fourth, we re-test in an effort to replicate results. When an attempt is made to scientifically evaluate acupuncture, it becomes difficult to apply all of these principles. This is because many psychological variables exist in acupuncture that are difficult to evaluate.

I recently heard a broadcast by a very reputable physician who said he is absolutely positive that acupuncture will not be effective in this country. It is effective in China only because people have been led to feel that the procedure must be valuable. Yet we know that many Caucasians have benefited from acupuncture, both here and abroad.

We also know that witchcraft is effective. In many countries, shamans and medicine men still practice folk medicine based upon belief systems that we do not hold sacrosanct. Yet their methods seem to work with many of their clientele.

Some time ago, here at the Postgraduate Center, we invited a psychiatrist from an African country, who was the son of a chieftain in a primitive part of that country. He had been educated in England both as a physician and as a psychoanalyst. His objective was to go back to the locale where he had been raised and bring scientific, non-magical psychiatry to the native population. He did so. And the results he reported were pretty much what could be expected. He found that he was practically completely ineffective. When a tribesman became depressed or developed anxiety or a phobia, he was much more likely to react favorably to a witch doctor, who diagnosed the type of spirit infestation and then prescribed appropriate rituals accepted by the group to be specifically designed for his trouble. However, when the doctor tried to apply what we would call scientific psychiatry to the problems of his people, it resulted in failure. There was no traditional acceptance of his methodology. The natives could not relate to what he was doing.

Do we have to make a similar situation with acupuncture? Although we have to examine matters more intensely and gather more information, preliminary investigations seem to indicate that acupuncture results are only partly related to belief systems. My hunch, corroborated almost daily by reports from Caucasian investigators, is that we will find acupuncture to be effective in people of our Western culture as well as in those of the East. Certainly if the reports of acupuncture working in animals are true, we can say that factors other than belief systems are operative.

Often we hear that acupuncture is a form of hypnosis. I have had many people write to me, inquiring: "As an authority on hypnosis, wouldn't you say that acupuncture is related to hypnosis?" My reply to them has been: "I don't know. Maybe it is, and maybe it isn't. In all probability there is some hypnotic influence in acupuncture, as there is in almost any kind of human, and particularly medical, relationship. But this is not the entire story. There are other things too."

What are these variables we have to consider in acupuncture? Foremost, as in any kind of procedure, we must take cognizance of the placebo effect. And this, as you know, is a very powerful effect. It accounts for a good number of the cures reported not only in physical but also in psychological medicine. One cannot avoid the placebo influence. It is a part of acupuncture, as it is a part of surgery, as it is a part of psychoanalysis, as it is a part of general medicine.

But is acupuncture solely a placebo? My hunch is no. But since the placebo effect is a part of the mosaic that constitutes any measure of pain relief, it undoubtedly is present in acupuncture.

Another hypothesis that has been presented is that acupuncture, psychologically, is nothing more than a relationship dependent on the bedside manner of the healer and the momentary positive and expectant transference that exists between healer and patient. You find the relationship factor in all types of healing. And we know that the bedside manner in medicine is a powerful therapeutic weapon.

Obviously, relationship is a factor in acupuncture. A person is ill; he reaches for some kind of an idealized, powerful authority figure who can eliminate his illness and bring relief to his suffering. This factor exerts an influence above and beyond the placebo effect.

But is acupuncture a relationship situation? Yes, in part; but not entirely. It enters into acupuncture only as one of the fragments that constitute its totality.

Another factor to be considered in acupuncture is "suggestion." The suggestive influence may be an important factor in Orientals, brought up to expect and anticipate that they will be helped by needles inserted in their skin. If a patient feels he is not going to be helped by being penetrated with needles, a negative suggestive factor is apt to occur, which will negate the positive influences that are operative. We must consider the latter factor carefully, since an individual on the basis of negative suggestibility can experience pain even though we would anticipate and expect that there would be an alleviation of pain.

We have some experiments in hypnosis that prove this point. When an individual has a stake in retaining pain for some psychological reason, he will not yield his pain. And this, I am sure, is going to occur with acupuncture, as it occurs with other forms of pain relief, even in the practice of anesthesia and nerve-blocking.

I remember one patient who came to me with very severe pain in his back. His orthopedic surgeon had prescribed a fusion operation since, in the opinion of the surgeon, the patient had problems in his back which could not be solved in any way other than by a fusion. There were additional opinions and contradictory reports from other consultants. Pharmaceutical analgesics had absolutely no effect. Other orthopedic procedures and remedies, including graded exercise, resulted in no pain relief. And so, in desperation, it was recommended that a fusion be done.

However, the patient's general practitioner thought that the possibility of a conversion hysteria should be eliminated. Hypnotic ablation of pain would establish it as functional and contraindicate operation.

Fortunately, the patient was a good hypnotic subject, and I found that it was possible to put him into a deep trance. What I did then was to suggest that the pain in his back would be transferred to his right arm. When he came out of the trance he would feel an excruciating pain in his right arm, but the pain in his back would be eliminated. Out of the trance, he straightened up and said excitedly: "My God, my pain is gone." He walked around the room. "But," he paused, "this arm is killing me. I can't raise it. What did you do to it? It's terrible." Having been in a somnambulistic state, he had no recollection that I had transferred the pain to the right arm.

This led me to believe that this symptom of pain was an hysterical phenomenon, that for some reason he had a stake in maintaining pain in his back.

I put him back into a trance and then transferred the pain over to his right leg. On awakening, he got up to walk around the room and almost fell down. He could hardly support his weight on his right leg.

I did the same thing with his left leg. My rationale was to teach him that it was possible through psychological means to transfer pain. I then shifted the pain to his left arm. When he came out of it, he exclaimed, to my surprise: "The pain is right back where it was before—in my back." I said, "Try to lift your left arm." He did. "Do you feel any pain or discomfort?" "No," he replied.

I then put him back into a trance and transferred the pain over to the right arm. This worked. I repeated the experiment with the left arm, but nothing happened.

This, to me, was very curious. So I enjoined him to engage in free association. I asked him to tell me about what the pain in the left arm meant to him. As he talked, he began to develop an emotional reaction. He talked about his father, who had died from a heart attack. Prior to this, his parent had experienced anginal symptoms with radiation of pain down his left arm. He revealed that he was afraid he had inherited his father's weakness and that some day he too would develop a heart attack.

This apparently explained why he absolutely refused to acknowledge pain in his left arm, because of the meaning of the location of such pain.

There are psychological reasons why some people have a stake in retaining pain. I am sure this will occur in a certain percentage of persons on whom analgesics, acupuncture, and other measures of pain alleviation will prove unsuccessful. A negative suggestibility factor plays a role in such denial of relief.

On the other hand, positive suggestion enters into the picture too. I once talked in front of a group of physicians about hypnotic anesthesia. There were some doctors present who were skeptical about the hypnotic phenomenon. One said he never could be hypnotized, even though a number of stage hypnotists had tried to put him into a trance. I asked the audience if there were any more people who had attempted it but were not able to be hypnotized. Two other doctors raised their hands. The three failures were then seated together in front of the audience. I instructed them as follows: "Would you mind closing your eyes. I don't want you to fall asleep. All I want you to do is to concentrate on your right hand. I'm going to stroke your right hand, and as I stroke your right hand just imagine that you're wearing a thick heavy leather glove."

I then stroked the right hand of each of the three doctors. They were fully conscious, but relaxed. Then I said: "Imagine now that you have taken your left hand and plunged it into a hot pail of water. Just visualize this. Visualize yourself plunging your hand into a pail of hot water, and then signal to me by raising your index finger when you see this." When this suggestion was followed, I firmly commented: "You'll begin to notice now that the left hand will be very sensitive, as if you plunged it into hot water. However, your right hand is going to feel as if it's got a stiff heavy leather glove on it. It will feel numb."

I then took a needle and went around and touched the left hands of all three. In each case when I poked the left hand even lightly, there was some hand withdrawal. I repeated this with the right hand, and no reaction seemed to have registered. When I asked them to lift their eyes, they looked at their hands and marveled that some numbness remained in the right hands.

This was done without hypnosis; just pure suggestibility in a state of relaxation. The analgesia was induced by relaxation and visualizing wearing a stiff, heavy leather glove. One of the doctors said he was positive that I did not use a needle in touching his right hand; he felt I was faking it. Had I used an acupuncture needle and told these subjects it would alleviate pain, I would predict that analgesia would occur.

Another important variable has to be considered in the investigation of acupuncture. This involves the doctor who does the acupuncture research as well as treatment. Does the operator have a conviction about what he is doing? Does he have faith in his work or doubts about its efficacy? Is he reasonably objective? An operator with negative faith or skepticism will have a desire to disprove a hypothesis. He almost unwittingly may do things to bring about negative results. Here is a story which accents this point.

Some years ago—many, many years ago—an experiment was done where an investigator depancreatinized a group of rats. He had a hypothesis that he would present a large array of food to the rats and that they would instinctually choose a diabetic diet, and this is exactly what happened. The rats selected food elements that substantiated the experimenter's hypothesis.

The experiment was reported in the press and was accepted at face value. Thirty-five years later or so the experiment was repeated by another investigator, with the same startling results. Again the depancreatinized rats selected a diabetic diet. The only difference was that our concepts of diet had changed, and the rats who apparently had been reading all the latest literature had selected items in the second experiment that they had rejected in the first.

Experimenter attitude and *experimenter bias* is something that must be considered in any research design. Moreover, the competence of the experimenter must also be considered. An incompetent professional may be suspected of achieving unreliable results. It is often not the method or instrumentality that is at fault; it is how it is implemented.

We find this in evaluating psychiatric methods. How often do we hear: "Well, I've experimented. I tried behavior modification with one patient and also psychoanalytical techniques, and I found that the behavior modification method worked better in this case and also in all of my other cases." Another person executing the same type of techniques will find universally that he gets nowhere with behavior modification, but his psychoanalytically-oriented tactics seem to bring results.

Again, bias, expectation, and the avidity with which the experimenter applies himself to the experiment, or the doctor relates himself to his patient, will have a profound effect upon the results.

What about hunches? Do I personally have a hunch about acupuncture as a form of hypnosis, the random product of non-specific variables? My initial impression in hearing about acupuncture originally was that it was a species of hypnosis. I do not think that now. While hypnosis may be a factor in acupuncture, I doubt that it is the principal factor. I have talked to a number of people who have studied acupuncture, and who have a conviction about the procedure. I have asked them all the same question: "Have you had experience with a sizable number of patients who have undergone major surgery?" In some cases the answer was, "Yes." "In terms of percentages, how many of this group have responded positively to acupuncture to a point where one could use acupuncture as the sole anesthetic?" The reply that I received ranged in the average of 80 percent.

Now, I do not know if this percentage is correct—some Chinese quote an even higher figure—but if it is correct and not based on hearsay, if 80 percent of people can be brought to a sufficient depth of anesthesia to do major surgery, I would say that this fact alone immediately eliminates the hypnosis hypothesis. *Only 10 percent can be brought to a depth of hypnotic trance sufficient to perform major surgery.* As far as minor surgery is concerned, almost all who can be hypnotized—which means most people—can achieve some skin anesthesia to allow some minor surgery.

The next question we must ask ourselves is: Is there an organic factor involved in hypnotic anesthesia, and does this factor apply to acupuncture anesthesia? There have been a number of hypotheses about what constitutes hypnotic anesthesia. Some of the physiological hypotheses are quite fanciful, such as a temporary dissociation of the synapses. Actually, it is my impression that what happens in hypnotic anesthesia is that there is an abatement of tension and anxiety because of the induced relaxation, and that through suggestion, attention is diverted. The pain threshold rises as a consequence.

Beyond question, in acupuncture there is a diversion of attention away from the pain area brought about by the acupuncture needles or electrical stimulation. There is an alleviation of tension and anxiety brought about by the patient's faith in the method. There is a bountiful expectation of cure, a healing factor in the relationship with the operator, a placebo influence, the powerful impact of suggestion, and probably a number of other variables that enter into a healer-subject relationship. But I doubt that these will explain everything we have to account for in acupuncture. There may be many other factors—perhaps physiological ones—that we now know little about, but which will undoubtedly be clarified with more sophisticated research and investigation.

[End of Dr. Wolberg's address]

Hypnotic Aspects of Acupuncture

As Year III of the Great American Public Acupuncture Experience draws to a close, it becomes more and more evident that the well-publicized Chinese medical curiosity, injected into the American mainstream more than 3½ years ago, is slated to occupy a permanent place in the therapeutic world.

We would have expected individual scoffers, who refused at first to consider acupuncture seriously, to be long since gone. Such is not the case. In fact, the modality is now faced with greater antagonism from semi-organized poor-mouthers trying to dispute it by insinuating it is something else—namely, hypnosis.

As a continuation of his right to freedom of speech, everyone is entitled to his opinion. There is, however, a tabu about hollering fire in a crowded theater. Falsely judging and labeling an entity that could eliminate 50 percent of our drug saturation problems is not a matter of a simple difference of opinion. It can only be classified as unfair and unscientific, and a freedom which is not granted. Why critics are so anxious to promote their unfounded assertions is incomprehensible. While supportive reports of beneficial results continue to arrive from every direction, their criticism seems to mount with total disregard for these findings.

In the beginning, there were individual "testimonials" from hundreds of American patients. Perhaps justifiably, these were ignored or ascribed to placebo or "Lourdes" effects. Fair enough. But later eyewitness reports were added by dozens of sober American physicians visiting in China. There were so many of them that their credibility could not be doubted. These were succeeded by individual testimonials from local doctors, just beginning to use acupuncture in their practices. Many of them produced daily "miracles" in their offices with just a few treatments. And concurrently, numerous scientific reports began to flood the newspapers, journals and scientific magazines. Somewhere along the line, the N.I.H. and several universities stepped in with some of their early reports.

But none of this satisfied the cynics. The gainsayers, provocateurs, and the putter-downers merely hustled extra hard to add their negative comments. It was almost as if some of them had a personal stake in seeing to it that acupuncture would never become established in this country.

Today, many more doctors feel the subject is over-the-hump as far as acceptance is concerned. The first N.I.H. acupuncture grant to the University of Missouri has been followed by research money to Columbia and New York universities. Others are sure to follow. More and more doctors are attending symposia and preliminary workshops that demonstrate how they can at least begin their preparation towards incorporating acupuncture in their practice.

And still the collective chorus of negative opinion has not diminished. It seems rather to have organized itself in some insidious manner, attempting to make inroads at the basic science level. Take, for example, this quote from the bulletin of one of the most prominent postgraduate schools of medicine in the city of New York. In a description of their regular curriculum courses on hypnosis, given by a competent, well-intentioned physician, the catalogue states: "Hypnosis is a technique . . . for understanding traditional clinical relationships, acupuncture, etc." It is interesting that this teacher can explain acupuncture so easily on a hypnotic basis when it is well known to aficionados that there is no real explanation as yet for hypnosis!

Another quote, this one taken from a widely circulated medical newspaper, states: "Acupuncture has been dismissed by knowledgeable hypno-therapists as part of the ritual ceremony induction we call hypnotism." What this statement implies, rather than what it says, deserves investigation. What are the boundaries of knowledge of a knowledgeable hypnotist? Does it mean that if one studies hypnotism for a number of years, one automatically, instinctively, knows about acupuncture without having to take the time or make the effort to first examine it most carefully? Apparently, in the case of knowledgeable hypnotists, this sort of preparation for a validated appraisal isn't necessary.

Negative statements in medical school catalogues and medical newspapers dismissing acupuncture as hypnosis seem to encourage a climate of stubbornness and closed-mindedness. Not too long ago —less than 20 years ago, in fact—"knowledgeable" physicians were dismissing hypnotism as outright quackery. The author remembers when the *JAMA* refused to publish even a simple letter to the editor which contained the word "hypnosis" because it might imply scientific endorsement. Let's not be too hasty with our dismissals.

Even if we include a growing number of Chinese-American M.D.'s, many of them having studied acupuncture in their youth, very few physicians are familiar with *modern* Chinese acupuncture technique. This type of acupuncture dates from 1958 in China, and some authorities claim it was preceded by "Ryodoraku" in Japan from about 1950. It must be distinguished from classical Chinese precepts which rely heavily on mnemonics, meridians, and unacceptable mumbo-jumbo. The ideology is very recent, built up in the Orient on a basis of advanced acupuncture thinking. Few classicists are aware of the electrifying of needles, and the applications to modern surgery or analgesia. Both the Chinese and the Russians claim it is definitely not hypnosis. And too many distinguished American scientists, most of them well-acquainted and trained in suggestive and hypnotic phenomena, are readily available to support this feeling.

We must not allow our colleagues of the loyal opposition to do the scientific community a disservice. Their verbal smokescreen and unscientific allegations will only slow mutual progress and hinder intensive examination and future explanations not only of acupuncture, but of hypnosis as well. This controversy is exhausting, wasteful, and should be prevented from creeping into our literature and our thinking. As we stated, it involves more than just a difference of opinion. At this point, we must get on with the research. If, in the future, after the research results are evaluated, it then becomes obvious that modern acupuncture is nothing more than a variation of suggestion, we are willing to stand corrected. But until then, we really must be allowed to get on with the work, and avoid useless, non-rewarding contention.

I take the following position: If there is a hypnotic element in acupuncture, it appears to be a corollary and not an essential part of the working mechanism. It has already been proven by early studies that there is only a casual relationship between the degree of hypnotizability and the effectiveness of acupuncture treatment in the same patient. Furthermore, the type of analgesia that acupuncture can produce cannot be duplicated by hypnotism, either qualitatively or quantitatively. Also to be considered are the rebuttals concerning the acupuncturing of children and animals, which have been heard frequently.

However, none of these arguments is as effective as this one simple test that has made believers of many skeptics: It is known by knowledgeable acupuncturists that without any preconditioning in a random patient, totally ignorant and uninstructed about either acupuncture or hypnotism, two acupuncture needles at Large Intestine 4 and two more at the Stomach 44 points, electrified, in 20-30 seconds can produce complete dental and buccal analgesia *selectively*. Hypnotism cannot duplicate this feat, nor can it ever begin to duplicate the other phenomena of acupuncture: the selective chest analgesia necessary for long lung operations; or the return to function of a patient suffering from glaucoma or deafness; or the multitudinous other phenomena produced routinely during acupuncture therapy. We know simple operations can be done with hypnosis alone, but with acupuncture the effectiveness of the analgesia is increased by many times, and the selectivity is remarkable.

It is time for the gainsayers to lay down their cudgels. Acupuncture, even if it contains elements of hypnosis, is one of the most important phenomena to appear on the medical horizon. While it cannot be equated with the discovery of penicillin, it nevertheless is deservant of more than the short shrift and dismissals it receives in some quarters. To paraphrase a remark made by James Reston, who once said, "There is something here too important to be left to journalists":

There is something here too important to be dismissed by hypnotists, or explained in terms of something like hypnosis—which can't be explained in the first place.

Only 27 years ago a physician I knew was overjoyed to find a communication from the then editor of the AMA *Journal*, George Halperin, which stated that despite the use of the word *hypnosis*, his paper would be published in the *JAMA* anyway. At that time the climate was not unlike what we find today with regard to acupuncture. Hypnosis was not at all well-defined at that time, and I wonder if in spite of much fine work since then it is any better understood today. There is no question that we know a good deal more about it, but the final analysis still eludes us.

So the argument whether acupuncture is or is not hypnosis seems rather simplistic. If it is hypnosis, then it is a very special kind of permutation and directly related to the type of acupuncture under discussion. It is definitely not subject to the same rules. It does not have the same statistics. People who cannot be hypnotized can get relief from acupuncture. People who have not been helped by hypnosis have been helped by acupuncture. Animals, who usually do not respond to hypnosis, are definitely helped by acupuncture.

For critics to isolate acupuncture and say it is nothing but hypnosis displays not only a poor foundation in the art itself but also a remarkable naivete regarding the therapeutic method. In a one-to-one treatment situation, it is an obvious contention that *all* therapeutic sessions contain elements of the hypnotic setting. This applies equally to everyday medical office visits of modern urban dwellers or tribesmen visiting their shaman. First, there is motivation: the patient wants to get well. There's an aura: the patient is impressed by the professional degrees and learning of the practitioner, perhaps by his office, perhaps by the bones hanging around his neck. And finally there is every probability of success, since the patient was quite possibly recommended by someone treated successfully by this same doctor. Three important elements in hypnosis.

Let us get back to the classification of the acupunctures and state that the degree of hypnosis varies with the type of acupuncture.

With classical Chinese techniques, there is mythology and demonology at play, and there is no question but that the suggestibility factor is high. There are talismen, secret recipes, and all the other trappings required of a mystical effect. Because of the generations of Chinese that have gone before, and who in illness turned to acupuncture as readily as we turn to the aspirin bottle—here, the hypnotic element is the probability of success. The individual has grown up with and seen so many people helped by acupuncture that a beneficial result is expected. However, this does not explain the large number of Caucasians who have had excellent therapeutic results. After all, a toothache is a toothache, and in my experience acupuncture can stop the pain immediately regardless of race, creed, or color.

Modern Chinese techniques involve a mixed bag of tricks, up to and including political motivation. So many patients undergo acupuncture treatments clutching the Little Red Book of Chairman Mao that it would seem impossible to separate the political element from the hypnotic precept. Quoting from the Peking Acupunctural

Association's answer to why acupunctural anesthesia works, they state: "We believe that so long as we study and apply Chairman Mao's philosophical thinking persistently we certainly can gradually understand, through repeated practice, the scientific truth of the theory of acupunctural anesthesia." Here we even see the principle of repetition, and if that isn't hypnosis, then what is it? But again, acupuncture goes beyond the normal hypnotic capabilities in so many instances we cannot attribute the results to that alone. And as someone has said, animals can be helped by acupuncture without ever having read Chairman Mao's book.

In acupuncture pain-blocking, the electrical techniques introduced eliminate most of the areas of hypnosis, since the application is based more on neurological principle than on suggestibility. Certainly suggestibility could play a part, but since the percentage of success is as high as 90 percent, it seems that it is not to be considered in this category.

We are fully aware that surgery can be performed on patients with only hypnosis as the anesthesia. I quote from the *New York Herald Tribune* of December 4, 1958, on a closed circuit program prepared by me for the New York State Society of Anesthesiologists:

> A thousand physicians watched a closed-circuit television broadcast of a surgeon removing a growth from the breast of a woman whose sense of pain had been eliminated by hypnosis.
>
> They also saw a motion picture of the removal of a thyroid gland under hypnosis without any ether or other anesthesia being used. Both operations were called successful.
>
> The breast operation was done at St. Vincent's Hospital as a demonstration for the New York State Society of Anesthesiologists' Tenth Post-Graduate Assembly. The physicians viewed it on a fifteen-foot screen at the Hotel New Yorker.
>
> Dr. William S. Kroger, Associate Professor of Obstetrics and Gynecology at Chicago Medical School, who mesmerized the patient, pointed out that only 10 percent of the population would be able to undergo major surgery while hypnotized. He emphasized, however, that it was a potent adjunct to chemical anesthesia agents to relieve tension and nervousness before major surgery.
>
> This, he said, does not reflect upon their intelligence, since mentally retarded or mentally ill persons usually cannot be hypnotized effectively enough for surgery. The more intelligent the person, he said, the better able they are to concentrate and produce the hypnotic state, as a rule.

> The patient who had the breast operation had been previously hypnotized at the time of the operation, Dr. Kroger said. He had only to instruct her to look at a spot in the ceiling to send her back into the pain-free condition.
>
> Then, by a series of instructions, Dr. Kroger made her lose all sense of feeling in her hand . . . this he called glove anesthesia. By asking her to touch her hand to her chest, the woman then lost all feeling in her breast. The operation then proceeded while Dr. Kroger kept assuring her and inducing her to fall into a deeper hypnotic state.
>
> After the operation Dr. Kroger asked her to come out of the hypnotic state. She had no memory of where she had been or that she had even had an operation. She had no nausea, pain or other discomfort.
>
> Dr. Kroger carefully pointed out that he had not developed the technique; it had been known even before ether was discovered. More than 100 years ago, legs had even been amputated under hypnosis. However, Dr. Kroger suggested a revival of the technique as an adjunct to chemical sleep induction.
>
> Actually, Dr. Kroger said, sleep and the hypnotic state were as far apart as the North and South poles. Hypnosis, he said, was an altered state of awareness. The patient can do only those things, he said, that the patient wishes to do, and Dr. Kroger added that as far as he knew there were no after-effects to this process.

This program, as I stated, was produced and directed by this writer, and the reason I mention that is that in the selection of subjects we had to choose patients who could be brought to the somnambulistic level of hypnosis before surgery could be started. The percentage of somnambules in the patient population is no more than 15. The Chinese are able to use acupuncture successfully in 90 percent. The truism to be learned from these statistics is obvious.

A final word about the way most American patients approach acupuncture, since it concerns hypnosis. It is totally unlike the faithful at Lourdes. There is little or no aura of faith or credibility; in fact, for most of them acupuncture is a last desperate maneuver. Mostly one sees the attitude "What can I lose?" rather than "I *know* this is going to help me." When acupuncture succeeds in these circumstances, there is something going on too important to be left to hypnotists.

To date, two definitive studies have been done on acupuncture and hypnosis, and another is about to commence. Dr. Ronald Katz, Professor and Chairman of Anesthesiology at the University of California in Los Angeles, after a study of 132 patients, has found a close correlation between hypnotizability and the degree of success with acupuncture. The author, in a study of 121 patients at the Postgraduate Center for Mental Health, has found only a random relationship between the degree of hypnotizability and the success achieved with acupuncture. Reports from various individual centers via personal communication have indicated that some of the patients who could not be hypnotized have achieved successful relief of pain with acupuncture. The reverse has also been found to be true, in that some people who could be hypnotized did not respond to acupuncture therapy.

At this writing, Dr. George Ulett, formerly Commissioner for Mental Hygiene for the State of Missouri, and Professor and Chairman of the Department of Psychiatry at the University of Missouri, is commencing a three-year study on this subject. He feels that, from early indications, it would seem that the hypnotic component is present in acupuncture therapy, but that the effect of the needling goes far beyond this. However, as a good scientist, he is reserving his final opinion until the data have been accumulated and interpreted.

CHAPTER IX

THE ACUPUNCTURE NEEDLE

From the beginning of its first historic day of usage, conflict and conversation have raged around which type of acupuncture needle should be used for what, by whom, and in which way. In fact, it is this degree of contention that led some wags to call the modality "arguepuncture." The controversy is not too different from the various combination acupuncture recipes which have been developed for treatment. Depending on which school you subscribe to, which countries you have visited, or which faculties you support, your acupuncture needle can vary widely, from a standard card of dressmakers' needles, purchased at the notions store, to gold custom-made needles imported from France.

There is no doubt that the type of needle and the technique of its insertion matter a great deal in the effectiveness of the treatment, but not as much as cultists would have us believe. Various materials have been used in antiquity, starting with bone splinters, dragon claws, and other mystical and magical items.

Bamboo and bone were in popular usage until metal began to replace them. Today it is generally acknowledged that stainless steel is the best material for the manufacture of acupuncture needles. If other materials are used, they can cause the deposition of harmful metallic fragments in deep-seated tissue, and give rise to foreign-body infections, abscesses, and so forth.

The stainless steel gauge usually preferred is between 30 to 32 French, or .3 millimeters in diameter in the mechanic's vocabulary.

The needle consists of several parts, the stainless steel forming the most essential part since this is the part which enters the human body. The needle should be manufactured so that it will not break and should be neither too long nor too short but exactly the right length for the purpose for which it is intended. Here we can discard the mysticism and rely on our common sense. If we are trying to probe a deep area, we use a longer needle. If we are interested in reaching superficial structures, then we use a short needle. Needles have been manufactured in lengths from one-half an inch up to eight inches, so there is a variety from which to choose.

The needle consists of four parts: the handle, the neck, the body, and the point.

Handles vary as widely as lengths. In some countries, practitioners prefer a thicker grip; in others, narrower. They will swear this characteristic makes it superior to other, thinner, handles, and results in better treatments.

Some are one piece and extremely thin, forming a collar over the body. Some needles, usually large in size, have a triangular point with triple edges, resembling a sail-maker's needle. They are used for blood-letting.

Other needles are grouped in clumps or clusters.

As a result of the embargo on acupuncture needles by the United States Government, a special needle with a handle has been developed that seems to offer several advantages in that it is easy to sterilize and literally screws itself forward, which helps considerably in needle insertion.

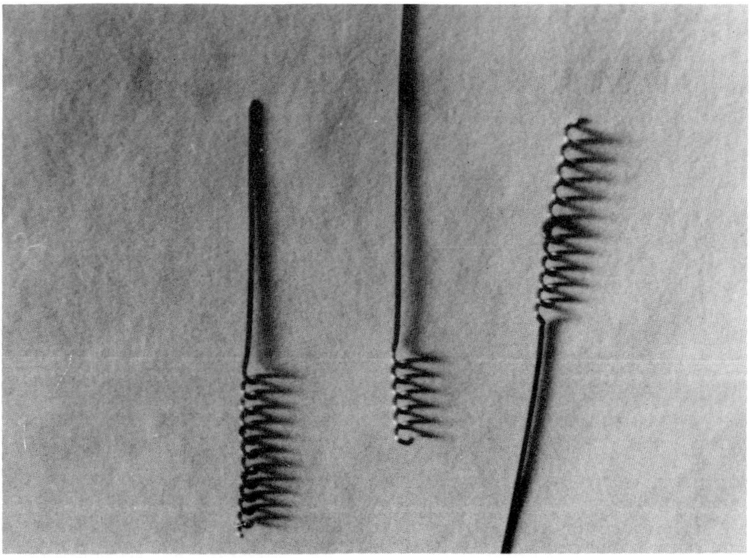

As in any needle, the point must be kept sharp. When a burr develops, trauma can be caused similar to the result of bending the point of our own hypodermic needles.

Much ado is made of the angle of insertion, and here again, common sense should be used. Mainly, the attempt should be to insert the needle as painlessly as possible and to provide a fair amount of needle imbedded in tissue.

A good trick is to press your thumb at the point of insertion for a minute or two before insertion, which gives a partial analgesia before the needle is inserted.

When working in or near the face, short needles should be used, since, obviously, deeper penetration will cause trauma to underlying structures. When working in areas such as the gluteal, where there is a muscular preponderance, you would use a longer acupuncture needle, just as normally you would use a longer intramuscular needle to reach the sciatic nerve.

Near the face and head, pinching the skin between the two fingers and pressing the needle into the raised fold of skin may facilitate insertion. In and about the ear, a sleeve, introducer, or "straw" may be used, which simply prevents the needle from bending as force is applied for insertion.

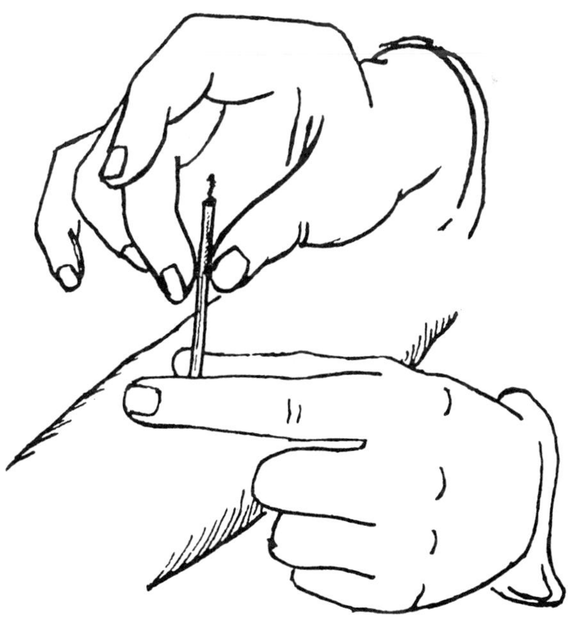

For longer needles, the fingers may also be used instead of an introducer, although this is considered taboo by Western practitioners because of their fear of sepsis.

Acupuncture needle insertion should produce little or no pain, and upon withdrawal should result in no bleeding. If there is anything we can learn from experienced non-medical acupuncturists, it is the agility and skill with which they are able to insert needles into the human skin and avoid these two major side effects of needle insertion. Practice on yourself with acupuncture needles. It will bring a new understanding to the task of how to do it properly on other people. In China, potential acupuncturists begin to practice on themselves and on their colleagues at a very early age. By the time they have reached graduation age, they are experienced and capable, and are able to insert the needles without either pain or ecchymoses. A residue of black-and-blue marks is the undeniable trademark of a clumsy acupuncturist, not inclined to improve his reputation or increase his referrals.

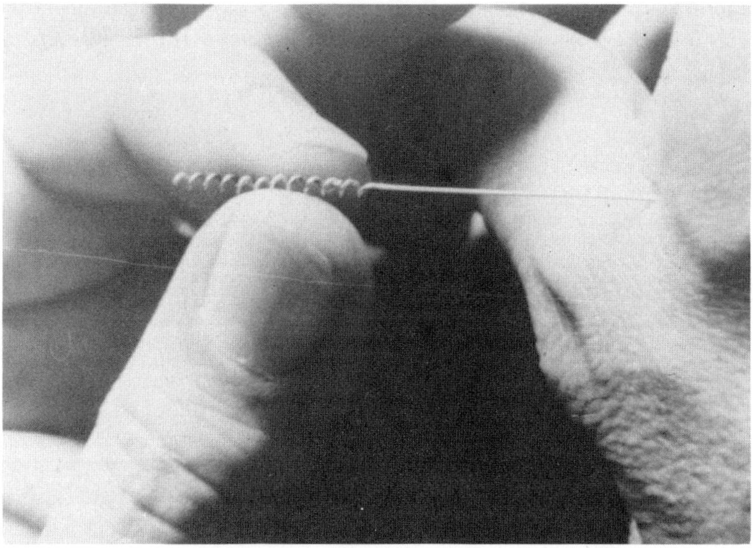

Needles of good quality stainless steel may be sterilized and used again. The needle illustrated above is manufactured at a cost which allows it to be used once and then disposed of, thereby avoiding the problem of any sort of cross-infection.

The average insertion of the acupuncture needle at the loci is not more than a half to three-quarters of an inch. However, deeper insertion is required in some instances. This is where the trained physician's knowledge of surface anatomy becomes indispensable.

At all times, there is no substitute for experience. Although the Chinese claim that needles can be inserted at three main angles—the right angle, 15-degree angle, and the 45-degree angle—experience has proven that these are not infallible and depend a great deal on whether the patient is erect, supine, prone, or in any other position; the acupuncturist's understanding of these angles; the force of entry; etc. The average Chinese patient does not allow too much examination or undressing. One realizes suddenly that acupuncture has been performed quite frequently through the clothes! This practice is inconceivable in Western thinking.

Dr. Chu Lien, a Western-trained Chinese, very active in acupuncture research in the Orient, is the practitioner who feels that the force of the acupuncture, and not the angle, is of importance. Others feel that the rotation should be clock-wise and not counterclockwise. Still other acupuncturists insist that the acupuncture should be performed with simultaneous stimulation of the front and back. Of such rules are religious dogma and acupuncture mythology created.

Our common practice when using the needle is to acupuncture bilaterally, in obeisance not only to the ancient laws of establishing the balance between Yin and Yang but also in deference to the sensory decussation. When following this law, one must be sure that electro-acupuncture is not contemplated. Placing needles bilaterally and connecting them to even the weakest electrical current (as weak as the EKG machine) is satisfactory if the wires do not cross the chest. When they do, it provides the basis for a possible fibrillation of the heart and even electrocution. Recent operating room studies have proven that passing the weakest electrical currents across the chest can cause serious arrhythmias and must therefore be avoided at all costs when using bilateral acupuncture.

The needle will affect patients in many ways, and it is important that we do not overlook the hypnotic aspects and transference which occur. Patients who have been accustomed to being put to sleep or sedated by the needle will get sleepy. Others who have used needles for stimulation, such as methadrine users, may develop a euphoria. Most frequently, patients describe a sense of tonification, which is the basis for its use in psychiatric practice. Others, with a high pain threshold and a long medical history, will state they did not feel the needle at all. Hypersensitive patients will complain even before they are stuck.

At the point of insertion, a localized erythema will sometimes occur. These patients will usually respond well to treatment (not a hard-and-fast rule).

An attempt should be made to produce a tingle—called *tei-chi*. It has been said that when this is achieved, the treatment will be most successful. It is reminiscent of the specialist in regional anesthesia, who probes for nerve before injecting the local anesthetic.

A more generalized or systematic effect of tingling or warmth is also produced, extending from areas or regions of the body to enveloping the entire body.

In electrical acupuncture, the needles are identical with those used for single-treatment acupuncture. In these cases, the necessity for using very high-quality stainless steel becomes imperative. Under the dissociation stimulation of electricity, an alloy which allows for the electrical separation of metallic ions will undoubtedly cause a chemical burn. One such case has been recorded personally, and others have been reported elsewhere, indicating that the electrical current was able to deposit copper ions deep at the site of the acupuncture; the healing process to eliminate this foreign corrosive material required eight to nine months and assiduous medical care.

Some world-prominent acupuncturists, such as Dr. Nguyen Van Nghi, insist that the larger the needle, the easier it is to induce acupuncture analgesia. Perhaps this is so, but it is also more painful. We have also seen severe small abscess formations which could only have been initiated by the increased tissue trauma initiated by inserting large needles.

CHAPTER X

USEFUL AREAS FOR DERMAL PUNCTURE

Chinese traditionalists insist that when the proper acupuncture point is not penetrated, they achieve very poor results. They proclaim that the acupuncture points, approximately 1/10 of a millimeter in diameter in most cases, must be known, located exactly, and entered in a particular way; otherwise the desired effect will not be forthcoming. In order to attain this mathematical precision, years of study are required.

In my experience, this has proven to be another romantic notion. Relief with acupuncture has been obtained in many instances merely by feeling for sore points or trigger points or trigger zones. If the pathologic condition involves a muscle bundle, the muscle bundle can be penetrated at several points. Even the Chinese know this phenomenon, thereby accounting for the large variety of combinations and recipes, all designed to cure similar maladies.

It is our contention that the average physician's knowledge of the course of mixed cutaneous nerves is more than adequate to treat most illnesses which are responsive to acupuncture. What he must be aware of is that he should not penetrate the nerve, but attempt to introduce the needle close to it. In this respect, the technique is very similar to that employed when doing a standard nerve block. To alleviate the pain of introduction, the needle should be inserted quickly so as to penetrate the outer layer. Once this is done, depth of insertion can be accomplished by screwing and advancing the needle at the same time. The specially designed American acupuncture needle enables this motion to be performed with ease, since the handle of the needle is, itself, threaded to resemble a screw.

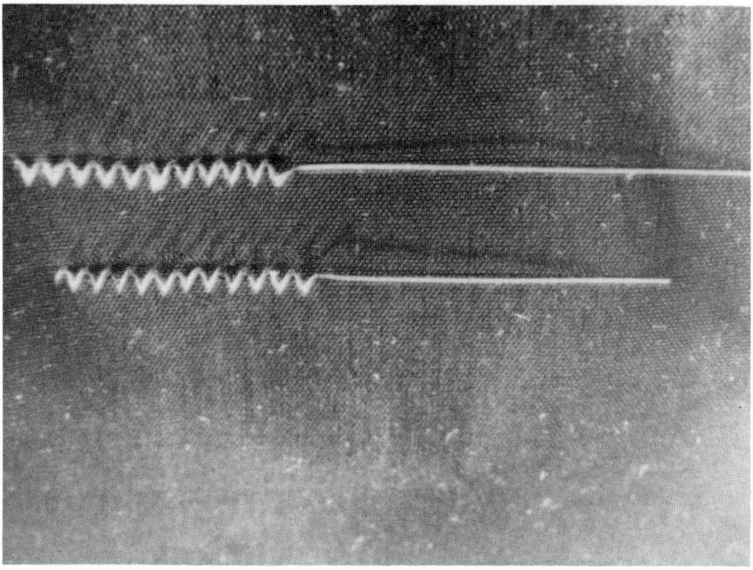

Great emphasis is placed by the Chinese on the angle of introduction. Interpretations of "stimulation," "sedation," "tonification," and other cultish ideas are attached to the angle of introduction. This, too, falls by the wayside in actual clinical practice. Suffice it to say that the angle of introduction should be such as to cause no damage to surrounding structures. When working in areas near the face, eyes, mouth, dome of the pleura, and so on, a profound knowledge of surface anatomy is essential. The bony and fleshy landmarks of any area must be thoroughly reviewed before attempting to needle. The rules of reasonable care and caution must be studiously applied at all times.

In essence, it can be said that acupuncture points, which form the basis for long years of study for some acupuncturists, need not be discarded entirely, for they most certainly teach us where we can stick a needle into the human body without causing too much damage.

For the benefit of those American physicians who are so steeped in traditional Chinese medicine that they cannot bear to tear themselves away from it, we will review some of the more common acupuncture points and then attempt to relate them to the nerve or neuromuscular bundle or neuro-vascular bundle which most assuredly lies in close proximity to that point. It must be clearly understood, however, that these points do not bear the same relationship to the effects produced as a telephone number to a telephone. Specifically, one does not merely look up a disease, see which points are listed, and then proceed to acupuncture those points, expecting a "cure" to be effected. Would that it were so! Not only the practice of American acupuncture, but world medicine would be greatly improved thereby.

Unfortunately, many volumes, in both their original Chinese forms and in their English translations, do adopt this approach. It is not true in the classical Chinese tradition, since they treat the entire individual and augment acupuncture with the other modalities found in Chinese medicine, such as moxibustion, herbs, massage, and diet. This list is delineated mainly to act as a teaching aid. Since most physicians already know the nervous system, relating the acupuncture points to this system will help them memorize some of the major points. Here are a few examples:

PATHOLOGY	ACUPUNCTURE POINT	NERVE
Headache	Lung meridian pt. #7	Radial
Hypertension	Kidney meridian pt. #1	Plantar
Toothache	Stomach meridian pt. #42	Peroneal
Lumbago	Bladder meridian pt. #54	Popliteal
Insomnia	Stomach meridian pt. #45	Medial & Lateral Plantar
Nosebleed	Governing vessel pt. #23 }	Supra Orbital
Hemorrhoids	Governing vessel pt. #20 }	Supra Trochlear
		Auriculo Temporal
		Temporal

These points follow an old Chinese custom in that they seem to be far away from the illness; and, in fact, it is frequently recommended that the points chosen not only be far away but also on the side opposite to the affliction. Add this to the list of notions which have been carried down through the years. If the point selected appears not to be effective, several other points along the course of the same nerve may be needled to increase the effectiveness. If it works, write down these locations and keep it to yourself, for you have just developed a secret acupuncture recipe not unlike the ones that acupuncture "families" boast of in the Orient.

To continue with our formulary of acupuncture points, we now come to the points which are utilized in conjunction with other points on differing meridians. For example:

PATHOLOGY	ACUPUNCTURE POINTS	NERVE
Upper G.I. tract problems	Large intestine meridian pt. #2	1st Digital (Median)
	Stomach meridian pt. #36	Peroneal
Lower G.I. tract problems	Stomach meridian pt. #44	Medial & Lateral Plantar
	Tri-heater meridian pt. #7	Post. Anterbrachial Cut. Post. Branch of Medial Cut. Post. Inteross. (Deeper)
Oral problems	Small intestine meridian pt. #7	Facial
	Stomach meridian pt. #4	Mandibular, Buccal
Esophageal problems	Large intestine meridian pt. #4	Ulnar, Radial
	and #11	Musculo-Cut., Radial
Nasal problems	Large intestine meridian pt. #4 and #11	(See Above)
Pharangeal problems	Large intestine meridian pt. #19 and #20 }	Labial, Facial Gt. Palatine
	Stomach meridian pt. #20	Intercostal 9 & 10
Otologic problems	Large intestine meridian pt. #4 and #11	(See Above)

Chinese acupuncture points are also classified according to diseases, and over the centuries a formulary has been developed which is very much like a dictionary of diseases, with a knowledge of proper acupuncture points allocated to that disease readily available. Here are some examples.

ABDOMINAL DISTENTION	**ST-36,25,44, C-12** (LV-1, ST-20) add LU-9, LI-11, VC-3,5,10,12 LV-13 (Extremities—Ton B-20, Sed. SP-9, B-23, K-7, Moxa VC-9) (Swollen, edema—Sed VC-6,11,17, ST-36) (Stomach full, regurgitation—Sed ST-25,44, VC-12, B-21, Ton. B-20) (Constipation, black stool—Sed. VC-3, SP-10, B-17, Moxa LV-13,14) (Pain, face hot, red, spotted—Sed VC-12, ST-44, Point one inch above SP-10) (Abdomen swells—Moxa VC-6, B-20,17, LV-13) (Feces, foul, abdominal pain—SP-4, P-6, ST-36, VC-12,4 ST-25)

	ADDITIONAL POINTS: (ST-44, LI-4, LV-4, ST-37, VC-9, ST-22, B-57, LI-8, SP-6, VC-12,13) (Irregular diet, sour regurgitation—Sed VC-12, ST-41, P-6, LV-3) (Sighing, bad breath—Sed VC-11, ST-36, ST-44) (Vomit contains mucous—Moxa VC-14,10, ST-40) (May vomit blood, black stool—Sed SP-6, B-17, Moxa LV-14) (Mental depression, thirst—Sed P-6, ST-43) (Loose stool, heat provides relief—Moxa VC-14, VC-4) (Weak, pressure provides relief—Ton ST-36, VC-6, B-20) (Aerocolon—K-8, ST-19,29, SP-6, ST-36, VC-8, LI-3, LV-3) **EAR POINTS**—STOMACH, SMALL INTESTINE, SYMPATHETIC, DIVINE GATE
ABORTION	**SP-6**,15 **LI-4**, B-60,31,32 VC-4,6 GV-2,4,3
ABSCESS	(Breast—GB-21, LU-7, B-54) add B-17, SP-10 (LU-7, SI-1, SP-18) (GB-41, LI-8, SI-34, P-7) (VC-17) (Cervix—VC-12) (Face—ST-2,3) (Liver—B-42, ST-40,45 GB-16) (Mouth—GV-27) (Scalp—B-4)
ACNE	See DERMATITIS
ADDICTION	**EAR POINTS**—LUNG, LIVER
ADENITIS	(Axillary—P-1,7 B-19, GB-38) (Cervical—T-12,22 SI-8) (Facial—LI-1,20) (Inguinal—ST-45, SP-11) (Inguinal blennorrhagia—ST-31, LI-1) (Knee—GB-30) (Lumbar—GB-30) (Maxillary—T-22, ST-5) (Popliteal—B-55) (Sub-maxillary T-22, LI-10) (Thigh—GB-30)
ADNEXITIS	**EAR POINTS**—UTERUS, OVARY, INTERNAL SECRETION, DIVINE GATE See PELVIC INFLAMMATORY DISEASE
AGALACTIA	After childbirth—SI-1,2
ALCOHOLISM	Psychiatric points (H-5,7 etc.) **EAR POINTS**—FOREHEAD, SUBCORTEX, BACK OF HEAD
ALOPECIA	B-54 **EAR POINTS**—LUNG, INTERNAL SECRETION, KIDNEY, OCCIPUT, C.P.
AMENORRHEA	**(LI-4, GV-2, VC-4, SP-6)** (VC-4,3, B-23) add SP-6 (B-37,38) add VC-4, ST-36 (LI-4, SP-6, B-38) (ST-36, 25, LV-8) (VC-3,2, ST-29) (B-60, VC-2, GV-1) (Surgery, trauma, insufficient flow—Ton. SP-6,10, VC-6, B-18,20,23) (Emotional upset—Ton. LI-4, Sed. SP-6,10,8) (Abdomen swollen—B-38,20,21) add VC-4, ST-36 (Abdominal pain—ST-29) (Constipated, distended—K-13) (Backache—Ton. B-23) **EAR POINTS**—UTERUS, INTERNAL SECRETION, OVARY ADRENAL, KIDNEY
AMNESIA	(B-15,23, VC-4, ST-36, H-7, H-3) (VC-12, ST-40, B-15, ST-36) (LU-7, H-7, P-6, K-1)
ANGINA PECTORIS	(Tone B-15, 1" deep; Sed. H-7, ¼" deep; Sed. ST-36, 1¼" deep thru P-6) K-23
ANOREXIA	(H-7, P-2, T-1) add K-27, T-1, GV-9, VC-9,12,14 SP-4,8,19,20 ST-20,21,22,23,36,37,39 42 GB-28, T-1, P-2, K-3,17,18,22,23,24,25,26,27 B-17,22,40,41,42,43,44 H-7 **EAR POINTS**—STOMACH, SMALL INTESTINE, PANCREAS, GALL BLADDER SYMPATHETIC, SPLEEN
ANURIA	(B-23, VC-6) (B-65,67) (Extreme urgency **K-1, VC-1**) (Special resuscitation points—VC-1,2,4) (Resuscitation of the drowned—VC-1, SP-9, ST-27, 28,36,40 LV-5,8,9,10 K-8) B-26,30,31,32,33,34,48,50,52,67 H-8 **EAR POINTS**—KIDNEY, BLADDER, SYMPATHETIC, EXTERNAL GENITAL ORGANS, SUBCORTEX
ANXIETY (Nervous with palpitations)	**H-7, GV-24, LI-4, P-7** (H-9, K-1) add GV-24, VC-14,17, LU-4,10, LV-2,5, GB-19, K-1,4, SI-7, P-2,5, H-5,6,7,8,9 (Children—LV-2) (SI-3, B-62) **EAR POINTS**—SUBCORTEX, DIVINE GATE, STOMACH, HEART, KIDNEY
APHONIA	(H-4,5,6,7) (GV-16, VC-23, LI-4) add T-5, P-5 (Hysterical aphonia—**K-1**, LV-1, LU-11, LI-10,18, B-10, VC-23, T-17, SI-15, GV-15, GB-12, LI-17,4, K-4, H-5) **EAR POINTS**—BRAIN STEM, OCCIPUT, FOREHEAD
APNOEA	K-27, ST-13,14 LI-3,4 GB-10, GB-40,41 K-25,27 **EAR POINTS**—SEE ASTHMA
APOPLEXY	VC-24, GV-16,20 LI-9,10, GB-3,39, T-10, P-5, B-54, B-62 See CEREBRAL HEMORRHAGE
APPENDICITIS	(X-LE-14, LI-11, ST-44,25) RX tid **EAR POINTS**—APPENDIX, SYMPATHETIC, LARGE INTESTINE, DIVINE GATE
ARTERIOSCLEROSIS	P-8, GB-34,39 ST-36
ARTHRITIS	NRG, SP-21, P-6 See **PAIN SYNDROMES**
ARTHRITIS, RHEUMATOID	ST-36,37,39,40, K-7, VC-2,10,22,23, NRG

ASCITES

(ST-45, SP-4, ST-43,45 GB-28) add VC-12,6 LV-13, B-20, VC-9, ST-28, SP-6, GB-28, K-7, ST-36, SP-6,9
EAR POINTS—STOMACH, SYMPATHETIC, SUBCORTEX, DIVINE GATE, LIVER

ASTHMA

LU-7, B-13, VC-16, LI-4

Acute attacks (cough) XBW-4, VC-22, XBW-8, P-6, VC-14, B-13, LU-6, ST-40 Leave needles 30 minutes twirling every 5-10 minutes daily

Mild attacks (debility) GV-14, B-13, ST-36, B-23, VC-4, VC-12, B-20 Stimulate 2-3 points q.o.d. Moxa points on back. Stimulate two bilaterally. Leave needles in 15-20 minutes. **Acu injections:** XBW-4, LI-4, Inject 0.1-0.2 ml. Adrenalin

LU-9,10, SP-3, H-8, NRG, **LU-5**, VC-17, inserted diagonally caudad 1½", use EAR POINTS. **LU-5**, acts like steroid.

(LU-9,10, H-8, SP-3, NRG, VC-17) (Insert VC-17 caudad, subcutaneously a distance of 1½" (LU-5, twirl 3-5 minutes—acts like Adrenalin) Additional points—ST-12, K-27, B-11,12,13,17 use **EAR POINTS P-VC-7, VC-22,21,16, B-31,33** (Between episodes, any 2 to 4 main points for treatment) (Treat daily 7-10 days) (VC-21,16, Acute attack—twirl 2-5 minutes) add LI-4, ST-36 (Moxa between asthmatic attacks) (Moxa GV-14, B-12,13)

(Emotionally upset, white thin sputum, bronchial congestion, non-productive cough—Moxa **B-13**, VC-12,17, LU-7, Sed. B-13, LU-7,11, VC-21, ST-40) (Chest congestion, can't breathe, skin dry, cough productive—Sed. B-12,13, LU-5, VC-17, ST-40, B-23,38, ST-36, VC-4) (Emergency during asthma attacks—Ton. VC-17, B-12,15, Sed. VC-22, ST-9, LU-7) (Sed. T-5, LI-4, Moxa VC-9, KI-23) (LU-7, LI-4, B-13) (Profuse yellowish sputum—ST-40, VC-22, LU-5) (Sweating & weakness—LU-9, B-13, ST-36) Ton. Moxa (Dyspnea on exertion—VC-6,17, GV-4, B-23) Ton. Moxa (Persistent cases add: B-17,43, VC-12, B-20)
Acu injections: XBW-4, LI-4, Inject 0.1-0.2 ml. Adrenalin
EAR POINTS—SYMPATHETIC, LUNG, GOD'S DOOR, CHECK DYSPNEA, ADRENAL, ENDOCRINE, DIVINE GATE—stimulate two bilaterally. Leave needles in 15-20 minutes.

BELL'S PALSY (LI-4, ST-4,6) (ST-4,6, B-1, T-17, LI-4, ST-44, LV-3) Rx affected side Moxa and alternate. Additional points—SI-18, GB-12, T-17, LI-4, ST-36, LU-9

BLENORRHAGIA (LV-1, VC-1) (Chronic—GV-1,2) (Chronic—GV-1, VC-1,2,3,4, SP-11,12, LV-1,3,4, K-4,6,7,8,10,11,18, B-25,27,31,32,33,34,35,48,57,61)

BLEPHAROSPASM ST-1
EAR POINTS—EYE, LIVER

BLOOD In expectorant—GB-44. See HEMORRHAGE, HEMOPTYSIS, HEMATEMESIS

BLURRED VISION See CATARACT

BOILS (On face—LI-1) (On nose—LI-20, GV-25) (In ear—T-21, B-65)

BREAST TUMOR GB-44. See MASTITIS

BRONCHITIS

LU-5, B-13, XBW-4, ST-36 (Chronic productive cough, pain in chest—Sed. LU-5,9, Ton. B-13, Moxa VC-17) (Dyspnea, coughing, chest and back painful—GV-12,10, B-13, VC-17, P-6, LU-5, VC-12, ST-36)
(Acute Bronchitis—B-13, LU-5, ST-40) if fever, add GV-14, LI-4 **(Chronic Bronchitis**—VC-22, vertebral points C-7 to T-6) Use 1-2 points, each treatment daily. (If Asthmatic—ST-40, XBW-4, CV-17 inserted 1½" subcutaneously caudad, ST-36)
Prophylaxis of Chronic Bronchitis—Moxa 2-3 points, every other day—GV-14, B-13,43, VC-6, ST-36
Acu injection—1 ml. of 1% Procaine in VC-22, daily for 5-7 days.

Chronic Bronchitis Gut Implant—XBW-4, VC-17, B-13, LU-6, ST-36
Additional points—K-27, LU-1, K-21,22,23,24,25,26, GV-10,11, VC-13,15,17,18,19,20,23, SP-18,20, ST-10,11,14, Chronic—ST-13, LI-8, LU-3,5, T-10, P-2,3, K-21,22,23,24,25,26,27, B-7,11,12,13,17,18,37,38,39, SI-15
EAR POINTS—ASTHMA-2, LUNG, ADRENAL GLAND, DIVINE GATE, BRONCHI

CARDIAC ARRYTHMIA (P-6, H-7)
EAR POINTS—HEART, SYMPATHETIC, DIVINE GATE

CARPAL TUNNEL SYNDROME (H-7, P-7, LU-9, P-6, T-5, NRG)

CATARACT (GB-20, B-1,18) add LI-4, ST-36 (Occasionally effective in early stage), X-HN-10, LU-9, LV-3, GB-1, B-8, T-1, B-1,67, GV-28, ST-6, GB-41, B-2, GB-14, ST-14

CEREBRAL HEMORRHAGE	ST-6,4, T-17, LI-4, LU-7, ST-36, GV-26, VC-24, GB-14, ST-2, GB-20 **EAR POINTS**—DIVINE GATE, ADRENAL GLAND
CEREBRAL ISCHEMIA	(GB-44, ST-45) (GV-20,21) (ST-37,39,45, LI-11) add LV-2, GB-44
CHOLECYSTITIS	1½" below GB-34, point approx. P-6 **EAR POINTS**—GALLBLADDER, LIVER, SYMPATHETIC, DIVINE GATE, INTERNAL SECRETION
CHOLELITHIASIS	B-18,19, GB-25,34, LV-14,3, VC-12
COLITIS	(ST-36, local points) add K-5, B-23, LV-11,2,8, ST-25,27, VC-12,4, SP-9, K-2, B-65, LU-9, B-54, LI-11, ST-36, SP-1, K-14,7, VC-9, B-35 **EAR POINTS**—LARGE INTESTINE, INTERNAL SECRETION, SYMPATHETIC, SMALL INTESTINE, DIVINE GATE
COMMON COLD	**GB-20, LI-4, K-7,**△ (Chills, fever, aches—GB-20, T-5, GB-12) (Fever, thirst, sweats, sore throat—LI-11,4, LU-5, T-5) **Add:** (Dry skin—Ton. LI-4, Sed. K-7) (Fever—Sed. GV-14, ST-43) (Headache—Sed. or bleed—GV-23, XHN-9) (Nasal congestion—LI-20) (Cough LV-7, LU-9) (B-12, LU-7, LI-4, GB-20, K-7, GV-16) Add: (Fever—GV-14, B-12) (Headache—XHN-9) (Stuffy nose—LI-20) (Cough—LU-5, B-13)—Treat daily (Prophylaxis—ST-36 daily for three days, or Moxa GV-14,13,12 daily, or rub GB-20 thirty times b.i.d. **EAR POINTS**—INTERNAL NOSE, ADRENAL FOREHEAD, LUNG. See BRONCHITIS, COUGH, LARYNGITIS, PHARYNGITIS, RHINITIS
CONJUNCTIVITIS	(GB-20, B-1, GV-22) (B-1, LU-9) (Severe: add LV-3, B-18,19) (Blurred vision: B-18,23) Ton., Moxa **EAR POINTS**—EYE, LIVER. See EYE
CONSTIPATION	**ST-25,36,44, LV-1, T-6** (LV-1, VC-1, LI-2) (T-6, ST-25) (Habitual—T-6, B-27,28,30,31,32,33,34,48,50,52,56,57) (Habitual—B-25,46, K-3,4,8,15,18) (Habitual—K-6, GB-27) (Habitual—GB-34, LV-1,2, ST-22,27,36,41, SP-3,5,13) (Habitual—SP-15, VC-1) (T-6, ST-25, B-25, GB-34) add VC-12, ST-36, LI-4, ST-44 (SP-6, B-57, VC-6, B31) (LV-13,3, SP-3, VC-12, B-57, K-6, B-23,24, K-15,16) (Weak abdominal muscles—SP-13) (Distended abdomen—B-28, Habitual constipation—T-7, GB-34, K-17,16, B-46) **EAR POINTS**—LOWER SECTION OF RECTUM, LARGE INTESTINE, SUBCORTEX
CONTRACEPTION	(C-5, ½" to 1½" deep—30 sec., LI-4, SP-6, Point 1" above medial maleolus rt. leg) RX q 3 days × 5 (Moxa for sterilization)
CONVULSIONS	See EPILEPSY
COUGH	**LU-7, B-13** (B-13, VC-22, LU-5, LU-7, PV-C-7) (Cough as in common cold—LU-7, LU-5, LI-4, B-13) Ton, Moxa (Due to bronchitis, pneumonia—K-3, LU-7, B-13) **EAR POINTS**—DIVINE GATE, ASTHMA-2, ADRENAL GLAND, BACK OF HEAD LUNG (Coughing, nose blocked, fever—GB-20, B-12, B-13) add T-5, LU-8, (Continuous cough, blood in sputum—B-37, B-38, GV-12) add ST-25, VC-6, ST-36 (Persistant—SI-1, K-1, LV-14) (GB-44, P-4, LU-2,6) (Obstinate—LU-8, LI-13,18, T-10, SI-11) add SI-2 (B-14, K-3, GB-8) (GB-10, GB-11,44 LV-14, ST-15,18,19,20) (ST-13, SP-5,14, VC-17) (Congestion, dripping sinus white sputum—Sed B-12, GV-16, LU-7, LU-9) (Fever, thirst, sore throat—B-12, B-13, T-5, LU-10) (Fever, thirst, sore throat, phlegm—LU-7, SP-5, SP-9, VC-12) (Hot, congested—B-12, B-13, LU-9, Ton K-7) (Anorexic, feverish, dry throat—Ton B-13, B-23, K-3, Sed LV-2, LU-5) (Anorexic, fatigue, pale—Ton ST-36, ST-40, B-13, B-20) **EAR POINTS**—ASTHMA-2, LUNG, ADRENAL GLAND, DIVINE GATE, TRACHEA SYMPATHETIC
CYSTITIS	(VC-4, VC-3, **B-23**, B-24, SP-10) add VC-6, SP-9, K-6, ST-28, SP-6 (K-7, B-54, SP-9, SP-6) B-26, B-27, B-28, B-29, B-30, B-54, VC-2, K-12, GB-25, ST-30, ST-31, LV-11, GB-1 **EAR POINTS**—URINARY BLADDER, KIDNEY, ADRENAL GLAND, SYMPATHETIC, DIVINE GATE
DEAFNESS (and Mutism)	**SI-19, T-17, GB-2, GV-15, LI-4, LU-7,** (NRG, VC-2,5,10, LI-11, T-2,3,5,16-21, GB-2,25, SI-19, ST-36, B-67,23, XBW-17a) Use electrical stimulation: connect T-5 to T-17 and T-21 to GB-2,—10 Hz, 10 minutes, 20 ua Frequency of treatment may vary daily, twice weekly, depending on ability of patient to follow thru with treatment. (T-21, SI-19, GB-2, GV-15, VC-23) add LI-4, T-3,5 (SI-19, T-17, B-19) add T-5, GB-43 (LI-4, GV-20, SI-19, T-17,21,3) (T-11, P-9, T-23, LI-1) (SI-19, GB-44, LI-1) (GV-20, GB-2, T-17, H-5, GV-15) add LI-4, ST-36, SI-19 (After illness or accident—GB-2, T-17, GV-15) add T-5, H-5

NOTE: Deafness which begins slowly and increases is not suitable for Acupuncture
EAR POINTS—KIDNEY, INTERNAL & EXTERNAL EAR, OCCIPUT, BRAIN, HEART, DIVINE GATE, THROAT, INTERNAL SECRETION

DEMENTIA LI-45, T-2,10, K-9, ST-23,45

DEPRESSION (H-7,9, GV-14) (H-5, ST-40, B-15, SP-1, LU-7,9) (H-9, LI-45) (Nervous—LI-4,11, B-10,22,38, GB-23, SP-6, VC-6, GV-8,13,18) (Fearful, insomnia, fatigue, cold in extremities: Ton. B-15,18, H-7, P-4) (Shallow breathing, Moxa GV-4, B-23,15, VC-4) (Chest congestion, productive cough: Sed. VC-9,12, ST-40, Ton. ST-36, B-20) (Insomnia, restless sleep, worry: Sed. H-7, B-15,19, P-4)
EAR POINTS—SUBCORTEX, DIVINE GATE, STOMACH, HEART, KIDNEY

DERMATITIS (**Acne Vulgaris**—LU-11, H-9, SP-2, B-54, LV-11, K-12)
(**Eczema of Hands**—P-8,6,7, H-8) (**Exzema, Weeping**—B-60,54, LI-11, T-5, SI-30, SP-10)
(**Folliculitis**—LI-11, B-54, SP-10, LI-15, T-5, LI-4)
(**Furunculosis**—LU-11, H-9, and deep breathing exercise)
(**Neurodermatitis**—LI-11, SP-10, LI-4, SP-6) Moxa
(**Pruritis**—LV-8, B-54,13, ST-15, GB-41, LU-7, GB-37,31, GV-20)
(**Psoriasis**—B-12, LI-11, T-5, B-54, SP-10, B-58, GB-31)
(**Purplish discoloration of face**—LU-9) (**Urticaria**—LV-5, LI-14, SP-6, ST-31)
EAR POINTS—LUNG, LIVER, ADRENAL GLAND, C.P., DIVINE GATE

DIABETES (Polyuria, Glucosuria, Polydypsia, Sed. B-13, LU-11,5, bleed points under tongue) (Polyphagia, weight loss, polyuria B-20, VC-12, ST-28,43) (Sed LV-2, K-2, Ton. VC-4, B-23) (Excessive drinking, micturition normal—B-13,15,21, VC-12, P-6, LU-10, K-3, ST-44) (Thirsty micturition immediately after drinking: limbs emaciated—B-15,23, VC-4,3, K-7, B-60) add LV-1, VC-24, T-4, B-20,23,28,29, K-2, LV-1,2 ST-33, GV-26

DIARRHEA **ST-25,36, SP-14,** (Chronic SP-15, VC-8) (Acute diarrhea ST-25,36, B-25, VC-12,6) add LI-4, ST-44,37, SP-9, B-25, (Chronic diarrhea—SP-6, B-20, LU-13, VC-12) Ton. add K-3, GV-4, VC-4, B-23, ST-36, GV-20, Ton. (Abdominal pain, watery stool light green—Ton. ST-25, VC-12,6, B-25) (Stool yellowish-red, anal burning, abdominal pain—VC-10, LI-4, ST-44) (Watery stool, no abdominal pain, stomach congested—Ton. VC-9, B-20, Sed. SP-9,4) (Wrong food indigestion, abdominal pain—ST-36, VC-12, B-21,25) (Abdominal gurgling, pain—Ton. ST-36, B-20,21, Sed. LV-2) (Feces dark, fatigue, slight abdominal pain—Ton. GV-4,20, VC-4, B-23,20) (Stools watery, abdomen painful—VC-12, ST-25, B-20,25,36,44, LI-11,4, SP-9, ST-39) (Belching, abdomen full—VC-13,12, ST-25, LV-13, P-6, ST-36,37,39) (GV-1, LI-3, T-18, B-20,25,26,27,28, K-16, ST-20)
EAR POINTS—LARGE AND SMALL INTESTINE, SYMPATHETIC, DIVINE GATE

DYSENTERY **(St-38,25, P-6, VC-4, LI-11)** (Emesis, fever—Intermittent twirling for 30 minutes—ST-38) (Treatment is 1-3 times a day) (Moxa VC-12, ST-25, VC-8,4) (Feces gummy, light, white jelly—ST-25, B-25, VC-10, T-6) (Feces red, thirst, fever, abdominal pain—LI-4, B-25,27, ST-44, B-41) (Feces white or red, anorexic, stomach full—Ton. B-20,21, Sed, ST-25, P-6) (Prolonged, recurring dysentery, difficult to cure, relieve temporarily—Ton.—B-20,23, Moxa, VC-4, Ton. GV-20, ST-36, Sed, ST-25) (Dysentery—ST-25, VC-6) add B-25,29, (VC-12, ST-25, LI-4) add SP-2, ST-44 (Trismus—B-20,21, VC-12, ST-25) (Dysentery LV-6, SP-6, VC-12, ST-36, 28,29, K-21, VC-6, T-5, P-6, ST-11, GV-1, K-7, B-62, LI-4, B-26, LV-2, SP-4) (pulse fast, fatigued—LI-4,11, ST-25,37,44, B-27) add B-20,21, VC-12, ST-36 (Rectal prolapse—GV-20)
EAR POINTS—LARGE INTESTINE, SMALL INTESTINE, SYMPATHETIC, DIVINE GATE

DYSMENORRHEA **VC-6,4, SP-6,4,** (B-23,47, GB-25, SP-6, NRG) add SP-1, LU-8, LV-1, ST-2, H-8, LV-4,8, K-10 (VC-3, B-17, VC-6,4) add SP-10, P-6 (VC-4, SP-6,4) (LV-8, LU-7, SP-6, K-3) (B-62, GB-35, LI-4) (ST-28, LV-14,16,15) (B-31,32,33) (B-34, GV-12) (Pain distention—LV-2, VC-6,3,12, SP-8) (Painful and irregular—SP-10, VC-4, LI-4) Moxa (VC-6, SP-6, ST-36, B-20) Ton. Moxa (**Severe**—Ton. Moxa—VC-4, Ton. B-23, LI-4, Sed. SP-6,10) VC-1,3,6,7, H-5, P-5, B-23,31,32,33,34, GB-26,29,41 (SP-1,2,6,13, LV-1,8, B-23,47, GB-25, NRG)
EAR POINTS—UTERUS, INTERNAL SECRETION

DYSPNEA (B-13,12, LI-4, LU-7,10) add T-5, VC-12, LV-14, LU-1, LI-1,20, SP-21, LU-5,7,8, LI-4,6,18, T-19, SI-15, B-17,20,37,39, K-3,19,20, K-25, GB-18,19,35, LV-14, ST-10,11,12,19, VC-15,16,18,20,21,22,23
EAR POINTS—SYMPATHETIC, ASTHMA-2, LUNG, ADRENAL GLAND

DYSURIA (Cystourethritis) (GB-34, SP-6, B-28,22) add GV-20, VC-4, Ton. or Moxa
EAR POINTS—URINARY BLADDER, KIDNEY, ADRENAL GLAND

EAR See OTITIS MEDIA & EXTERNA, DEAFNESS, TINNITUS

EDEMA	**SP-6, ST-36, VC-4**
Abdominal	(Ton. B-20, Sed. SP-9, B-23, K-7, **Moxa** VC-9)
Ascending (begins in feet)	(Ton. B-20,23, ST-36, **Moxa** VC-6,9) (SP-6, GB-34,39, ST-36,41, VC-4) (GB-31, SP-4,9, GB-30, B-54,57,58,62) (Generalized weakness, legs cold, painful—Ton. SP-6,10, K-3, GB-39, ST-36, B-58, VC-4) (Pain in feet and knees—SP-6, GB-34,39, ST-36,41, VC-4)
Cardiac	(SP-6, T-7, VC-5)
Face	**VC-24, LV-8, K-7, LU-1,** (VC-24, GV-26, LV-8) (T-16, B-20,45, K-7) (LU-1, ST-45) (Sudden swelling in face goes to upper extremities—LU-7, SP-9, K-7, B-28)
Generalized	ST-15,45
ELBOW	LU-11
EMOTIONAL INSTABILITY	(Worried, cries easily, emotions vary widely—Sed. P-7, H-7, Ton. B-15, K-1) (If severe—Sed. GV-20,26, LV-3, ST-14, P-5) **EAR POINTS**—SUBCORTEX, DIVINE GATE
ENDOCARDITIS	**SP-4, P-5,6, K-2,** SP-21, H-4, P-2,7, B-13,16,17,39,42,43, K-3, GB-41, SP-21
ENTEROCOLITIS	(Acute—GV-1,15,5, VC-6,10) (Chronic—VC-5,8,9,13, GV-3,11) add SP-1, B-17,22,25,27,29,35,41,48, K-8,14,15, ST-37 **EAR POINTS**—LARGE AND SMALL INTESTINE, SYMPATHETIC
ENURESIS	K-10, VC-4, SP-6 **EAR POINTS**—URINARY BLADDER, SUBCORTEX, BRANCH, KIDNEY
EPIDIDYMITIS	(Pain, low back, scrotum—VC-6, LV-2, SP-6) **EAR POINTS**—TESTIS, DIVINE GATE, EXTERNAL GENITAL ORGANS
EPILEPSY	(B-15,13,20, GV-14) add ST-36, P-6, GB-13 (LU-7, SP-9, K-7, B-28) (Spasm, fainting, foaming at mouth—Ton. B-15,18, K-1, Sed. ST-40, VC-14) add VC-6,9, (Ton. B-20,23, ST-36) **Psychomotor** (GV-12,26, VC-12, H-7) add P-5, ST-3,40 (GV-16, B-15, GV-26, VC-12) add P-5, ST-40, SP-6 (GB-20, GV-14, B-15, H-7) (P-5, SI-3, ST-40, LV-2) add VC-24, GV-1, K-19, T-12, SI-2,3,5, B-5,11,15, GB-36, ST-24,41,42, SP-4, VC-24, GV-1,6,8,12,19,20,26,27
EPISTAXIS	**LI-4,20, LU-11,** (LI-4, GV-23,14,16) (GV-14, Moxa, B-20, LI-20, GV-26, XHN-2, B-64) (CV-4, ST-36) (LV-5, SI-1, B-18, GV-24) (GV-20,15, LI-19) (GB-20, B-10, LI-11,10) (LI-4, ST-44, VC-4, B-54) (ST-36, SI-2, LU-3, GB-39) (B-64, LV-1) H-6, P-4,8 LU-3, LI-2,6,18, SI-3 (Children—GV-18,12,14,15,16,22,23)
ERUCTATIONS	LU-8,10,P-6, LV-14, GB-25, LV-13, SP-16, VC-12, SP-2,4 **EAR POINTS**—STOMACH, SMALL INTESTINE, PANCREAS, GALLBLADDER, SYMPATHETIC, SPLEEN
ESOPHAGUS SPASM	B-38, VC-17, SP-6, B-17, K-21, B-45, P-8, GB-20, B-18, VC-22, LI-11, SP-5) (Stricture—B-15,17,19) **EAR POINTS**—STOMACH, SMALL INTESTINE, PANCREAS, GALLBLADDER, SYMPATHETIC, SPLEEN
EYE DISEASES, OF	**All Conditions—B-1, GB-20, LI-4, Add for: (Conjunctivitis & Keratitis—**XHN-9) **(Glaucoma—**GB-14, XHN-9) **(Optic Neuritis & Nerve Atrophy—**ST-1 lat, ST-1) Treat daily for 10 to 15 days—resume after resting one week (Atony of eye muscles ST-4) (Blepharitis—T-10, ST-36, GB-3, SI-4, LI-2) (Blepharospasm—ST-1) (Blurred vision—nerve lesion?—Ton. B-23, 18, K-3, then Ton B-1,2, GB-16, 37,14) (Color Blindness—GB-1, B-1, GB-2,37, ST-36,2, GB-16, Ton. K-3, B-23,18) (Cysts on lids—SI-7)
	(Conjunotivitis—T 12,23, SI 6, B 1,67, K 11,12,13,15,20, GB 1,16 ST 43) (Inner Canthus—GB-15, GV-28, B-65) (Outer Canthus—GB-43) **(Conjunctivitis—**bleed LU-11, XHN-9—with headache add LI-4, GB-20, GV-23) **(Conjunctivitis—**B-67, T-23, GB-1) add B-1, LV-2, LI-4, GB-37 (T-5, LI-4, GB-3, ST-8) (GB-20, B-10, GB-14, SI-18) (ST-44, GB-15, T-3, B-1) (T-23, LV-2, P-8) (Fatigue GB-20,14, LV-8, GB-3, ST-1, B-2,1, P-2, GV-19 B-10, GV-24,5, LI-4, K-1, ST-8, GB-16, T-23) (Film over eye—SI-1, B-1,67, T-1,23, GV-28) add LI-4, T-2,3,20, SI-3, B-2,6,67, K-14,19, GB-15,40, GV-23, ST-1,2,3,
	(Glaucoma—GB-20, LI-1, K-1, B-62,8,ST-43, GB-3, GV-24, ST-3)
	(Keratitis—GB-1, ST-1, K-11,17, GB-1,40, ST-3) **(Herpes Zoster**—B-2, ST-2) (Lacrimation—excess or deficiency—ST-1, GV-28, B-2,18, GB-15) (K-15, B-15, P-7, GV-20, ST-8, GB-37, SI-3) (Myopia—B-9, ST-3,4) (Night blindness—Ton—B-18, GB-37, B-1, T-23, B-23) add GB-1,14, B-2,18,20, ST-1) (Photophbia—GB-20,13,15, LV-3, B-6,60, SI-5) (Pruritis—B-1, ST-2) (Scotomas—LV-2,14, LI-4, SI-4, GB-20,19,18,3, B-2) (Purulent—ST-8) (Spasm of ocular

muscles—ST-4,5) (Strabismus—Circumorbital points) (Weak vision—GB-1, LI-4, SI-6,15,8, GV-25,27, GB-16,17, P-2)

FACIAL PAIN (ST-1,4,6-8, on unaffected side, ST-44, to sedate) See PAIN SYNDROMES

FAINTING (Traumatic coma) Ton. GV-26

FATIGUE (Overindulgence—Ton B-13,20,23,38, ST-36, VC-4) (Back pain, loss of weight, vomiting blood, fever, sweating—Ton. B-13,20,23, SP-6, K-3, Sed. LU-5, LV-2) (Coughing up phlegm—Sed. ST-40, VC-22) (Fever, sweating H-8, GV-14) (Vomiting blood—LU-10)

FEVER **H-9,** B-5,19, ST-43 (After chill—H-9,6, T-6, GB-16,22,26, GV-16) (Intermittent—LI-1, H-2,8, LU-3, T-4, B-64, GB-41, ST-25,43,44, GV-23) (Nocturnal—GV-12) (Tropical—LU-1, Without sweats—P-9, LU-6, GB-6)

FLATULENCE **GB-25, SP-5, ST-36,**16,20,37,43, K-12,19, SP-7

FLU See COMMON COLD

FOLLICULITIS LI-11, B-54, SP-10, LI-15, T-5, LI-4

FRIGIDITY **VC-3, SP-6, B-23, K-12** (VC-3,4 SP-15,6—30 minutes weekly, 5-6 weeks) add B-23,22,32, ST-36 (NRG, VC-3,4, B-31) (VC-4,6, SP-15,6, B-22,23, ST-36) (H-7, LU-8, P-7) (Moxa B-23, GB-4, Ton. VC-3, SP-6) (Mental exhaustion—Ton. B-15,20, H-7, VC-3, Sed. SP-6, ST-40) (Fear, Fatigue—B-18,19, Ton VC-3) (Resistent—SP-6, "Sperm Palace", VC-3, B-23)
EAR POINTS—EXTERNAL GENITAL ORGANS, UTERUS, SUBCORTEX, INTERNAL SECRETION, KIDNEY

GASTRO INTESTINAL DISEASE (P-6, ST-36) add VC-12, B-21 (Ulcer—Moxa—VC-12, ST-36—between attacks of pain) (Dyspepsia—VC-12, ST-25, VC-6, ST-36) add B-20,23, P-6, SP-6 (ST-36,25, VC-13) (XLE-3, LI-11, ST-36) (Acid base imbalance—K-5, LU-9) (Spasm B-62, LI-4) (ST-36,34, VC-12, P-6, LV-13, ST-44) (With vomiting and distention—VC-6, B-20, SP-4, Tone then Sed. and Moxa) add LV-3, LI-14 (Pediatric digestive disorders—PIPJ)
EAR POINTS—STOMACH, INTESTINES, GALLBLADDER, DUODENUM, SYMPATHETIC, DIVINE GATE, ABDOMEN

GASTRITIS (B-20,21, VC-12, LV-13, ST-36) add P-6, LU-5 (Vomits mucus, coughs—B-17, VC-21, LV-13, VC-12) add ST-28, SP-9 (Globus hystericus—LU-3, VC-14, SP-17, VC-12, H-5) (Epigastric pain—ST-45, SP-4,13, ST-36) (Poor digestion—LV-13,14, SP-15, ST-36, GB-25) ST-45 (LV-8, GB-40) (VC-12, VC-3,10, ST-25,36) (B-17,22,41-45, GV-6-9) (Indigestion—ST-36, SP-4, LI-4, B-21) add SI-45, B-21, 22,42,43,44, K-20, LV-13, SP-5, (Pain around umbilicus—VC-8, Moxa) (Pains in lower abdomen—SP-6, VC-4)
EAR POINTS—STOMACH, SMALL INTESTINE, PANCREAS, GASSBLADDER, SYMPATHETIS SPLEEN

GOITRE (ST-10, LI-4) add GB-21 (Local points, T-10) **Toxic Goitre:** (With palpation of the heart—P-6, H-7) (With Heavy sweating—LI-4) (With swollen eyes—B-1,2, ST-2, GB-20) (With high blood pressure—GV-20)

HEART, DISEASE OF (see ENDOCARDITIS MYOCARDITIS **H-7, P-6, B-15** (**All affections**—K-1,23, LU-1,2,4, B-15,39,64, GV-11, VC-15) (Dilatation—SI-1, GV-44, H-7, ST-11, B-14,17) (Paralysis—B-13,17) (**Palpitations**—VC-4, B-15, H-5, P-7, ST-36) add H-7, VC-7, P-6 (H-7, P-6, H-5, B-15,23) add P-7, ST-36, GB-35, ST-41, H-3, K-24,25, Vc-12, LV-13, B-10, GB-20 (**Tachycardia**—H-5, GV-14, GB-20, B-10, LV-2, B-39,13) (**Hypercholesterolemia**—LV-2) (**Cardiac asthma**—H-9, H-4, SI-14,15, LU-1,2, GV-17, VC-18) (**Anemia**—B-38, ST-36, LU-9, SP-5) (**Arrythmias**—B-17) add P-6, H-7
EAR POINTS—HEART, DIVINE GATE, OCCIPUT

HEART ATTACK **Special Formula—emergency points H-7, GV-26.** **Angina**—Ton. B-15, (1" deep) Sed. H-7, (¼" deep) Sed. T-5, (1½" deep) into P-6.

HEAT STROKE (Light case—LI-4, LI-11, GV-14) (Severe—GV-26,20, B-40) (If not aphasic —add VC-23, H-5)
EAR POINTS—OCCIPUT, HEART, SUBCORTEX, ADRENAL

HEMATEMESIS (B-17,18, SP-1, T-5) See HEMORRHAGE

HEMOPTYSIS (B-17, SP-4, VC-12, B-13,43) Ton., Mx.

HEMORRHAGE (Cerebral—VC-8) (Ocular—P-6) (Intestinal—GV-1, B-17,18,23,25,34,35,55, SP-3,4,16, VC-4,6) (Stomach—VC-1, GV-1) (VC-12,19) P-7 (Postpartum H-7) (Stomach—B-15,18,20,23,24,27,49,50,5,57,58)

HEMORRHOIDS	**VC-1, GV-1, SP-10, B-57.** (VC-1, GV-1) add B-23,24,27,49,50,56,57,58. (Bleeding—B-54,60) (Chronic—B-35) (Bleeding—K-7, SP-5) (Bleeding—SP-6, VC-1, GV-1,2,4,6,20) (External without pain, swelling or color: Ton. GV-20, ST-36, B-24,35) (External, red, swollen, painful—Sed. B-25, ST-37,25, SP-9) (GV-1, ½" to 1" deep, insert needle on each side of point of coccyx; Sed. SP-10, 2" deep, GV-20) [Bleeding Hemorrhoids—(moist and itchy, bleeding with stool) Sed. GV-1, B-57, SP-10, **Miracle Points,** forearm, 4 inches above flexure of wrist, palmar side. One inch deep each of two points either side of ulna. (Two white points.)] (GV-1, SP-10, B-57, VC-20) **EAR POINTS**—RECTUM, LARGE INTESTINE
HEPATITIS	(B-18,19, ST-36, LV-3) add GV-11,14, T-17, GB-34 (Pain—hepatic or splenic area—GB-40) (Abdominal distention—SP-6, VC-6) (Fever—GV-14) (Impairment of liver functions, elevation of transaminase—B-18 thru B-19) (Elevation of icteric index—GB-34, GV-9) (Depression—T-17) Rx—daily in acute stage. **Acu injection**—Inject 0.2-0.5 ml. Vitamin B-1 or B-12, into two points—T-6, B-21, ST-36) **EAR POINTS**—SYMPATHETIC, DIVINE GATE, LIVER, EYE-1,2
HERNIA	(Sed. LV-1, SP-6, VC-6, Moxa VC-4, K-6) (Muscle hernia, trauma, penis swollen, painful, discharge—Sed. LV-1, SP-6, VC-6, Moxa ST-30, GB-34, K-3) (Hard swelling in lower abdomen—Sed. VC-3,6, LV-3, SP-9) (Hernia—LV-3, SP-6, VC-6, LV-12, VC-12) LV-1, B-27, K-6,11,14,16,17,19, GB-24,27,40, LV-1 (Scrotal—LV-12, ST-22,23,27,37,43,44, SP-3, VC-9,13, GV-4) (B-23, VC-4, LV-3) add SP-6, K-6, ST-29, SP-9, LV-2, ST-36, T-5 (VC-3, P-6) add LV-8 **EAR POINTS**—UPPER ABDOMEN, SUBCORTEX, INTERNAL SECRETION
HICCOUGH	(B-20,21, VC-12) add ST-25,36 (B-38,17, VC-17,6) add ST-36.
HIVES	SP-10,6, LI-11,4, GB-31 (Itching LV-8)
HYPERSALIVATION	LI-18, B-41, K-18, GB-23, ST-39
HYPERTENSION	(**Group 1.**—LI-11, LV-3) (**Group 2.**—GB-20, ST-36) add X'HN-10, X'HN-4 (Tinnitus, temporal headache, frontal headache—T-18 (Insomnia—H-7) (Two main groups alternately used) **1.** LI-11, ST-36, **2.** GB-20, LV-3. Alternate (1) and (2) each treatment 30 minutes daily. (Headache—X'HN-4, X'HN-9) (Insomnia—XHN-22, H-7) (Palpitation—P-6) **Acu-injections 1.** LI-11, ST-36, LV-3, Inject 0.1-0.2 ml. "Reserpine" solution into two points. **2.** ST-36, P-6, LI-4. For each treatment use and alternate one point each from upper and lower limb. Inject 1 ml. of 0.25% Procaine daily for 10-15 days. (Hypertension—LV-14, B-19,24, GB-25, LV-13, B-19,24, GB-25, LV-13,14) (Hypertension—Ton. K-3, B-15, Sed. LI-4) (Worry, headache, dissiness, insomnia—Sed. LV-2,3, Ton. K-3, B-15,23) (Cholesterol elevated, pain in chest, numbness extremities—Sed. ST-40, VC-12, LV-2, B-18, P-7) **EAR POINTS**—ANTI-HYPERTENSION, SYMPATHETIC, GOD'S DOOR, HEART, ANTI-HYPERTENSION GROOVE
HYPERTHYROID	H-7
HYPOTENSION	Ton. B-15, SP-6
HYSTERIA	H-1,4 GV-26, P-6, LI-4, K-3, SP-6 **EAR POINTS**—SUBCORTEX, DIVINE GATE, STOMACH, HEART, KIDNEY
ILEITIS	ST-27,36, B-21
ILEUS (Paralytic)	(ST-36, P-6) (ST-36, B-21) (VC-22,17, LV-4, CV-6) **EAR POINTS**—SMALL AND LARGE INTESTINES.
IMPOTENCE	**SP-6, VC-3, B-23,** (NRG, CV-3, LV-11,16) add K-11,16, B-31, LV-8,4, K-10, LU-8, (VC-4, SP-6) add B-23, ST-36 (B-38,18,23, GV-3, VC-4) (ST-36, SP-6, GB-34, LV-3) (B-20, LV-13, LI-10, VC-11, P-6) (LV-5,3, ST-36,28) (SP-9, K-7, LV-2) (K-10,2, LV-4,1) (ST-30, SP-6, VC-6, GV-4) (K-3, LU-7, K-12, VC-2) (Lack of desire—K-7, VC-4,7,1, ST-29, SP-6) (Pain low back, headache, fatigue, mental strain, Moxa B-23, GV-4, Ton. VC-3, SP-8) (Ton. B-15, 20, H-7, VC-3, Sed. SP-6, ST-40) (Fear, palpitations, restlessness, fatigue, Sed. B-18,19, Ton. VC-3) **Special formula**—SP-6, "Sperm Palace" VC-3, B-23. **EAR POINTS**—EXTERNAL GENITAL ORGANS, TESTIS, SUBCORTEX, (In women—UTERUS)
INFLUENZA	See COMMON COLD
INGUINAL PAIN	ST-45, SP-6.

INSOMNIA	**H-7, SP-6, LV-10,** (VC-13,12,10,6,3, GB-20) (GV-24,5, Point 2/3 between B-10, and GB-20) (H-7, SP-6) add P-6, SP-1, K-3 (Palpitation, lack of appetite—add B-20,15) (Irritability, dizziness, tinnitus, sore back—add B-15,23) (Fullness in epigastrum, sighing—add B-21, ST-36) Moxa (Headache, pain along ribs, bitter taste—add B-18,19) (Worry-tone SP-6,10, H-7, B-17) (With G-U symptoms—Tone K-1, B-23,15, Sed. P-8) (Anger—Sed. B-18,19, LV-3) (Stomach upset—B-21, VC-12, ST-40, P-6) (Weak, pale—Ton. SP-6,10, H-7, B-17) (Dizziness, backache, leukorrhea—Ton. K-1, B-23,15, Sed. P-8) (Headache, pain sides, short tempered, bitter taste—Sed. B-18,19, LV-3) (Stomach heavy, cough, constipation —Sed. B-21, VC-12, ST-40, P-6) (Insomnia—H-7, SP-6, B-15,20) add H-6, SI-3, VC-4, ST-36, (H-7, SP-6,9,1, P-6) (B-62, GB-41, LU-9, ST-36, T-19) (ST-27, B-13,30, GB-17, LU-1) (LU-9,10) (LU-11) ST-45, H-7, P-7, LI-4, K-6, GB-12, LV-2, **Special point—LV-10,** ST-27,45, SP-6,7,9, GV-4,18. **EAR POINTS**—SUBCORTEX, DIVINE GATE, OCCIPUT, KIDNEY.
INTERCOSTAL NEURALGIA (Myositis)	P-7, SI-5, LI-1, GB-38,44 (Right side—P-6, SP-17) (Left side—GB-40) (Left ribs painful, pain does not move—LV-14,13, B-17, B-18, add P-6, LV-4) (Right ribs swollen and painful, pleuritic rub—LV-14, B-18, VC-12,17, LU-1,9, LI-4, B-13,17, LV-13, VC-17, GB-41, ST-36, SI-5, T-6, B-62, K-1, B-36,41, 12 thru 17) **EAR POINTS**—THORAX, DIVINE GATE, OCCIPUT.
INTESTINAL PARASITES	(ST-36,44, VC-12, B-25) also point one inch above SP-10, "Nest of 100 Worms."
INTESTINAL OBSTRUCTION	(Tone B-20, VC-6, ST-36, SP-4) (VC-17,14, B-21,41, T-6) (SP-6, B-57, VC-6, B-31)
ISCHEMIA	see PERIPHERAL VASCULAR DISEASE
JAUNDICE	(VC-12, ST-36, GV-9, B-19) add GV-14, GB-34, ST-44, SP-4 (LV-8, GB-21, B-44, P-7, K-5, SI-14, ST-44, K-7) (LI-4, LV-4, VC-12) (SI-8, GB-38,40, SP-5, LV-8, B-38, SP-10, B-54) (Whole body orange-yellow color, chest painful to touch—Sed LV-3, B-43,19, SP-9, VC-11) (Skin dark yellow, no fever, fatigue, sweating diarrhea—Ton. B-23,20, VC-12, ST-36, Sed. B-18) K-1, P-6,8, LI-1, B-13,18,19,20, LI-16,17,19, GB-24, LV-13, ST-20, SP-5, GV-16,27,14. **EAR POINTS**—SYMPATHETIC, DIVINE GATE, LIVER EYE 1,2 GALLBLADDER.
JAW	(Swollen—LI-1) (Recurring dislocation—ST-7) (Inflammed—ST-6) (Mastication difficult—ST-6)
KIDNEY DISEASE	(B-23,47, K-3) K-5, B-54,22,24,62, VC-3, ST-36, SP-14, GB-24,25 **EAR POINTS—URINARY BLADDER, KIDNEY, ADRENAL GLAND,** SUBCORTEX, DIVINE GATE, SYMPATHETIC. See URINARY TRACT
KNEE PAIN	**ST-34, SP-9, GB-34** (ST-33,34,35, tender points) add H-8, SI-2, B-66, K-2, EAR POINTS ST-34, SP-10,9, GB-34, ST-36, SP-6 (Knee joints red, swollen, painful—ST-34, SP-9,6, K-7, LV-2) **EAR POINTS—CORRESONDING PART.** See PAIN SYNDROMES
LARYNGITIS, PHARYNGITIS	(Throat swollen, red, irritated, sore—bleed LU-11, T-1, Sed. T-5, VC-21, LU-5, LI-4) (Chronic cough, throat painful, hoarseness—Ton. K-6, K-3, LU-9) LI-1,2, K-7, VC-22,18, GB-10,11,12,13 (SI-19, K-1, LU-6, LI-17) **EAR POINTS—THROAT, HEART, DIVINE GATE,** ADRENAL GLAND.
LETHARGY	**GB-34, LI-11, NRG** **EAR POINTS**—SUBCORTEX, DIVINE GATE, STOMACH, HEART, KIDNEY
LUMBAR	(GV-2-14, B-11,20,21,22,23,25,27,48,54,60)
MALARIA	**GV-14, SI-3, T-5,** Use acupuncture and Moxa for slight sweating, shivering. Use only acupuncture for excessive, sweating, little shivering. Treat 2 hours before attacks. (Severe cases only—P-9, LI-11,13) (Malaria—GV-14, GV-13, P-5,6, LI-11, ST-36, GB-34) (Treatment should be 2-3 hours before each episode of chills) (Intermittent Fevers, Remittent Fevers, Malaria—GV-13, P-5, T-6, SI-3, GV-16, LI-4,11) **EAR POINTS**—SUBCORTEX, INTERNAL SECRETION, LIVER, ADRENAL, SPLEEN
MASTITIS	SI-1, P-1, LI-8, SI-1,2, K-3, GB-41, GB-42,43, ST-18,34, SP-12,18, VC-17
MELANCHOLY	H-9 See DEPRESSION
MENIERE'S DISEASE	GB-20, P-6, T-18, SI-19, ST-36, VC-12, LI-4 (Nausea—ST-36, and VC-12) (Hearing—T-18, SI-19) **EAR POINTS**—SUBCORTEX, INNER EAR, STOMACH, OCCIPUT, FOREHEAD, DIVINE GATE
MENINGITIS CEREBRAL	K-1, P-6 **EAR POINTS**—KIDNEY, BRAIN STEM, OCCIPUT, DIVINE GATE, HEART, STOMACH, SUBCORTEX

MENOPAUSE (SP-6,10, VC-4) (H-7, LU-9) (LV-1, SP-1) add SP-10,6
EAR POINTS—UTERUS, OVARY, INTERNAL SECRETION

MENORRHAGIA (K-14, VC-3) (VC-4, SP-6,4) (B-20, VC-6, LV-13) (LV-13, VC-6,3) (SP-6, ST-33)
EAR POINTS—UTERUS, OVARY, INTERNAL SECRETION, KIDNEY, ADRENAL

MIGRAINE See PAIN SYNDROMES, HEADACHE (LI-4, GB-20, GV-24, GB-14, LI-20)

MILK (Insufficiency after childbirth—P-1) (Insufficiency—ST-18, SP-18)

MOUTH All problems—ST-42,44,45. (Bitter taste—GB-38, LV-5, ST-36) (Dry—LU-5, GV-28, LV-8) add GB-44, LI-3 (Gingivitis—ST-24, H-9, P-9, LI-4, VC-24,23, K-2,9, GV-12, T-5, GB-41) (Hypersalivation—LI-18, B-41, K-18, GB-23, ST-39)

(Lips inflammed, cracked—ST-4, LV-3, LI-4, T-5, GB-41) (Lip spasm—ST-5) (Muscle atony—LI-1, ST-45) LI-1,2,) B-7 (Risorius atony—K-20) (Spitting blood—GB-33,34)

Stomatitis—LI-1, K-3,4, B-13, (LI-4, ST-36, B-15,20) (VC-24, H-8, SP-2, XHN-2, right hand side, Swallowing difficulty—K-21) (Thrush—B-15,23, VC-24, LI-4) B-27 ST-36, K-6, B-20 (LV-2, P-8, K-6) (Tumor—LI-7) (Ulcerated—LI-7)
See DENTISTRY

MYOCARDITIS P-9,3,4,6,7, T-6 See HEART, DISEASE OF
EAR POINTS—HEART, SYMPATHETIC, SMALL INTESTINE, DIVINE GATE, OCCIPUT

NAUSEA & VOMITING (ST-36, SP-4, P-6, VC-12, B-20, LI-13) Ton. Sed. Moxa (Fever, thirst—add P-3, B-40, Sed.) (Occurs after eating—add LI-3) (VC-12, LV-13, B-20,21) add ST-36, SP-6, LV-8,14, B-62, GV-12, P-6, B-17, P-5, LI-11, SP-5, SI-3, LU-7, LI-4, P-8, SI-1, LU-9, P-7.
EAR POINTS—STOMACH, SYMPATHETIC, DIVINE GATE, SUBCORTEX.
See VOMITING

NECK (GV-2,14,16,20, GB-21, SI-15, GB-20)

NEPHRITIS LV-14, T-9, B-22,23,25, K-13, GB-25,28,29, LV-14, ST-24,25, ST-28, VC-3,4,13.
EAR POINTS—URINARY BLADDER, KIDNEY, ADRENAL GLAND, SUBCORTEX, DIVINE GATE, SYMPATHETIC.

NEURALGIA
- Abdomen, lower—B-28,53, ST-26
- Arm—LI-11,12,14, LU-3, T-3,6,14, ST-16,17,18, B-37
- Arm, anterior—LU-9, SI-1, LU-13,15, T-7,8,9
- Axillary—GB-42, B-40
- Back—B-5,50, GB-27
- Calf—(Special point—GB-37) B-53
- Chest—LV-3, LU-4
- Cranial—GB-7
- Dental—VC-24, ST-3,7, GB-3, B-14, LI-2,5,6
- Dorsal—B-27, B-45,65
- Dorso-lumbar—GV-2,8,9, B-13
- Elbow—P-6, LI-10,11, T-5,1
- Epigastric—GV-5, P-6, ST-23, VC-15
- Face—ST-3,4,6, H-3, B-4,9,59
- Fibular—(Special points) GB-35,36
- Foot Dorsum—GB-42
- Forearm—T-1
- Frontal—H-2, ST-8, GV-23,24, B-2
- Genital—B-47
- Inguinal—ST-45
- Intercostal—GV-9,11, VC-15,17,21, GB-22,25,43, K-21-27, H-1,9,23,48, H-1,9, K-27, SP-21, LU-2,8,9,13-18,23,36,41, H-2,3,4,8, SI-1, LU-13, T-6, LV-2, ST-12,15,16,18,19,39, SP-17,18,20,21
- Knee—ST-35
- Limb, lower—ST-32,34,42, SP-6, LV-6, K-8, GB-39,
- Limb, upper—ST-7,9,13,14,
- Limbs (four)—LV-8
- Lumbar—B-22,23,24,25,26,28,29,49,50,60,66,64
- Lumbar region—GB-27, GV-1, K-7, GB-25,29, LV-3,1
- Maxillary—GB-7
- Neck—ST-6, GB-7, T-10, GV-16,28
- Ocular—B-9
- Occipital—T-12
- Popliteus—B-53
- Radial—LU-8
- Sacral—B-27,28,30
- Scapula—LU-8, GB-25,27, ST-13,14,16
- Sciatica—B-29, B-30,31,32,33,34,35,49,50,51,60
- Scrotal—VC-7
- Shoulder—B-5
- Shoulder posterior aspect—LU-2, LI-2,3, B-36,37
- Teeth, lower—ST-5,6, T-8,9
- Teeth, upper—SI-18
- Thigh—B-59
- Thigh, inner muscles—LV-8
- Trigeminal—B-7, GB-1, ST-6, GB-11,14, LU-7
- Uterine—LV-1, GB-26,27
- Uterine, post partum—VC-3

NEURASTHENIA GB-34, LI-11, NRG T-17, H-7, SP-6, XH-3, GV-20, P-6, VC-12, ST-25, VC-4, B-32, ST-36
EAR POINTS—SUBCORTEX, DIVINE GATE, STOMACH, HEART, KIDNEY.

NEUROPATHY ST-40,45, VC-15

NOCTURNAL EMISSION Restlessness, face red, and feverish: B-13, H-7, LV-3, K-1, (Chest feels dry, thirsty—VC-3, SP-10,6, K-3) (Fatigue—Ton. VC-3, VC-6, GV-20, B-23)
See SPERMATORRHEA

NOSE (Boils—LI-20, B-47) (Inflamed—B-3) (Polyps—B-4, LI-20, GV-28, LI-19,

	T-22, GV-20,21,23,25) (Rhinitis—△, ST-45, B-67, LI-20, GV-28, B-7) (Sense of smell impaired—LI-20, K-22,23,24) (Nostrils blocked, stuffy—SI-2, B-67, GV-23,25,28,△) See RHINITIS, SINUSITIS
NYMPHOMANIA	SP-20, ST-30,29, LV-2, K-3, GB-43
OBESITY	SI-19, ST-36 **EAR POINTS**—MOUTH & LUNG, (Use surgical stapel) for oral compulsives. Use STOMACH & LUNG for stomach oriented patients.
OSTEOPOROSIS	SP-6, B-57 **EAR POINT**—PARATHYROID
OTITIS EXTERNA	**SI-19, T-22, GB-2** (GB-1, ST-19, LI-4,11) (SI-19, LI-1) add ST-7, GV-4, GB-44. **EAR POINTS**—KIDNEY, INTERNAL & EXTERNAL EAR, INTERNAL SECRETION
OTITIS MEDIA	(GB-41,3, SI-19, T-21) (SI-15, ST-36, SI-3, T-15) add T-23, GB-1, LI-4, T-18,19, GB-20, T-17, GB-2,12 **EAR POINTS**—INNER EAR, KIDNEY, INTERNAL SECRETION
PAROTITIS	(GB-20, LI-4, LU-7) add T-17, T-5 (LU-11, LI-7,10,19, T-17, ST-5) **EAR POINTS**—PAROTID, INTERNAL SECRETION
PELVIC INFLAMMATORY DISEASES	(VC-4, SP-6, ST-30, LV-5, SP-10, ST-36, SP-9, B-20, SP-4, ST-30, LV-5) (Irregular & low—ST-36, SP-9,10) (Cramps—SP-4) **EAR POINTS**—UTERUS, OVARY AND THE HORMONAL SYSTEM.
PENIS	(Pain in, SP-6, ST-29, LV-2) See under URINARY
PERICARDITIS	P-1,6,7, B-13,14,16,17,40, VC-14 See HEART, DISEASE OF
PERIPHERAL VASCULAR DISEASE (Ischemia)	K-2, SP-6-7 same side, K-6, B-54 (Upper extremities—H-3, LI-11) add IDMC GB-34, SP-9 (Lower extremities—IPMT, Moxa acupuncture points. Treatment is indicated for intermittent claudication and Raynaud's Disease. (Cold feeling in elbows—H-1) (Epigastrium—GV-9) (Belly—SP-9) (Lower limbs—SP-1) (Knees—St-32) (Lower limbs—LV-4) (Nucha—T-15) (Limbs after fever—K-3) (Fingers—H-3) (Knees—B-31,32,33,34) **EAR POINTS**—INTERNAL SECRETION, ADRENAL
PERITONITIS	LV-14, SP-1, LI-13, B-29,63, K-7,8,17, LV-2,13,14, ST-20,36, SP-1,9,14 chronic—SP-10, VC-3,6,11,13, GV-9
PHARYNGITIS	(Acute onset, headache, fever, profuse sputum, difficulty in breathing, pain on indegestion—LI-1,4, ST-44) (Low grade fever, intermittent pain in throat, dry red, swollen—K-3, LU-7) (Soreness—**LI-17**, SI-19, B-10,19, K-6,1,2) (Dry—LI-6) (Pharyngitis, Tonsillitis—LU-11—let blood) add (LI-4, GV-16, LU-5, XHN-2—both sides let blood) add T-1, LI-1—let blood add T-5, VC-22, T-2, LU-10, K-3, ST-36,44, GV-16 (Tonsillitis—K-5, LI-4, SI-17, L-3, LI-9, B-12, VC-22, ST-40) (Pharyngitis—L-9, LI-6, GB-20, B-17,18, SI-14, ST-9,10, VC-22,23, T-16,15, ST-6,5) (Lack of taste—SP-5,4, ST-44) (Cervical adenitis—B-38, SI-8, GB-41, T-5,10, H-3, LI-14,13, ST-12, VC-17, P-1, LV-3, SI-17, LI-4, LU-11, LI-11)
PLEURITIS	H-9, K-27, GB-44, LV-14, LI-1, SP-21, H-3, LU-5, LI-11, T-6,14, SI-4,14,17, B-11,12,17,19,38,42,43,44, K-3,19,22,23,24,25,26,27, GB-22,35,36,40,44, LV-14, ST-12,13,14,15,16,18,40, SP-4,17,19,20,21, VC-13,14,18,19,20 **EAR POINTS**—LUNG, THORAX, INTERNAL SECRETION, ADRENAL.
PNEUMONIA, TOXIC	**EAR POINTS**—ADRENAL GLAND, INTERNAL SECRETION, BILATERAL
POST-OP PAIN	(ST-37, ST-25, LI-11) Rx for 30 minutes to 2 hours, repeat q 6-8 hours.
POST-OPERATIVE PROBLEMS, GENERAL	(Muscle tension, cold extremities, fever) LU-11, GV-16,14, B-60, LI-4, Ton. SP-10
PROLAPSE OF RECTUM	(GV-20,6, VC-8, GV-1, B-13,25) (VC-8, GV-1, B-24, ST-25,36) (VC-17, ST-25, B-24, ST-36, B-20,21) (B-25, ST-25,36, SP-6) (B-58,57, K-5, B-62) (GV-1,4,20) (SP-4,12, ST-15) (ST-25, P-6, T-7,3) add B-31-35 See PROLAPSUS
PROLAPSUS	(Uterine—K-1) (Uterine—LV-1) (Rectal—ST-8) (Rectal, sudden—VC-8) (Rectal—GV-6,20) Special point for all ptoses—**GV-20**
PROSTATITIS	(Urine hot, congestion lower abdomen—Sed B-23,28, VC-3, K-7, SP-9) (Fatigue—Ton. VC-4, GV-20,4) (Can't urinate, vomiting, abdomen distended, pulse irregular, condition serious—Sed. SP-10,6, B-47,54, Ton. K-1) **EAR POINTS**—PROSTATE, INTERNAL SECRETION, KIDNEY, BLADDER, OCCIPUT
PROSTATIC HYPERTROPHY	B-67, K-3, VC-2,4, SP-9, VC-3, SP-10

PRURITIS (Eyes—B-1) (Vulva—H-8) (Eyelids—LI-3, SI-3) (Vulvar—K-2,10, LV-8,11) (Perineum—SP-10) (Inner corner of eyes—GV-28) (General—LV-8)
EAR POINTS—LUNG, ADRENAL GLAND, DIVINE GATE, LIVER, SUBCORTEX.

RAYNAUD'S DISEASE See PERIPHERAL VASCULAR DISEASE

RECTAL BLEEDING (Blood visible before stools—B-25, GV-1, B-57,35) (Stools visible before blood—SP-1, ST-36, B-27, (Moxa) SP-6) (Hemorrhoids—B-58,57,54, GV-1, B-35, B-47,49, LV-8, P-7, SP-5, GB-39, K-5,8,10, B-50, GV-20, B-60)
EAR POINTS—LOWER RECTUM, SUBCORTEX

RENAL COLIC B-23, SP-6, B-47, K-3
EAR POINTS—KIDNEY, URETER, DIVINE GATE, SUBCORTEX
See "URINARY" CATEGORIES

RESTLESSNESS H-9, (And fear in children—LU-5)

RHINITIS △(GV-24.5, LI-20) (LI-4,20, GV-14, H-7, LU-9, B-1, GB-1,14,20) (GB-20, GV-23, LI-20,4, GB-30) (LI-4, LU-7, GB-1, B-2) (LI-20, GB-20, GV-14) (GV-16,20,28) (P-8, SI-2, ST-3,45) (T-17, GB-15,19) (Sinusitis—K-8, LV-8, GV-26, ST-7,1,3, GB-14, B-2, GV-28, B-64, ST-45,40, SI-1,18, K-3, B-62, LI-11,17,20, GV-23, B-12, GB-20) (Anosmia—SP-4, LU-9, B-3,4,1,56,60,17, ST-12, LI-20,19, GV-25,16, B-10) (Hay Fever—LV-8, K-9, LI-19, GV-23,16, B-10,11,12, VC-17,20) (Sneezing—LU-5, GB-4, ST-8, B-12) (Nasal polyps—LI-20,19, GV-28,26,25,14,15,16, K-3, LU-7) (Rhinitis—Alternate 1. and 2., **1.** LI-20,4, B-7, ST-40, **2.** Sed. GB-10, 34,39, LV-2) (XHN-2, LI-4, LI-20)
EAR POINTS—INTERNAL NOSE, INTERNAL SECRETION, ADRENAL, FOREHEAD, LUNG, DIVINE GATE

SCHIZOPHRENIA Group 1: **GV-26, LI-4,** LV-3, Group 2: XH-3, P-6, SP-6, additional points: GB-15, GV-14, GV-13, SI-19, B-1. Treatment once or twice daily using the two groups of main points alternately. Twirling continuously or intermittently for one half hour. If no response is noted in a week's time, additional points are added.
EAR POINTS—SUBCORTEX, DIVINE GATE, STOMACH, BRAIN STEM, HEART, KIDNEY

SCIATICA GB-30, B-50,51, trigger points, B-54,57,23, GV-3
EAR POINTS—SCIATIC, DIVINE GATE, OCCIPUT, BUTTOCK, ADRENAL

SHOCK K-1, P-6
EAR POINTS—ADRENAL, HEART, OCCIPUT

SHOULDER (To place arm behind back—SI-10,11,15) Additional points—LU-2, T-10,11,14, LI-14,15

SINUSITIS **LI-4, B-2, GV-23, T-23,**△ (Point ½ inch below the lateral zygoma, GB-31, LI-4)
See RHINITIS

SPEECH IMPAIRMENT (GV-15, VC-23) See DEAFNESS—MUTISM

SPERMATORREA (Nocturnal emissions—B-15,23, VC-4,3) add H-7, SP-6, K-12, B-38, ST-36 (SP-6, VC-4,3, ST-36) (ST-25, B-31,32,33) (B-34, K-23, B-47, SP-9) (B-67, K-12) add GV-1, B-22 (Nocturnal, in dreams—B-38,47, K-11,12,13, SP-6, VC-2,3,4,6,7, GV-1,4)
EAR POINTS—SUBCORTEX, INTERNAL SECRETION, TESTICLE, KIDNEY, DIVINE GATE, EXT. GENITALS

STERILITY (Female—K-1,2, VC-3, SP-6, P-3) (Male—K-11,12,13, SP-6)

STOMACH ULCER (ST-36,25, VC-13)
EAR POINTS—STOMACH, SYMPATHETIC, DIVINE GATE

STOMATITIS LI-1, P-8, LI-7, Ulcerous—SI-5 See **MOUTH**
EAR POINTS—MOUTH, INTERNAL SECRETION, DIVINE GATE, TONGUE, ADRENAL, SPLEEN, OCCIPUT

STROKE (Suddenly lose consciousness, teeth clenched, face red, no involuntary excretion of urine or feces—first bleed all 12 terminal points on fingers. Then Sed GV-20,26, LI-4, (1" deep) ST-6,40, Ton. K-1)
Hands flaccid, moisture gurgles in mouth, excretion of urine or feces, sweating—Moxa VC-4m, VC-6, Ton. K-1, ST-36, SP-6, VC-12)
Hemiplegia—(Unaffected side, Ton. LI-4, LI-11, LI-15, GB-30, GB-31, GB-34) (Affected side, Sed same points. Add local points in area of paralysis)
(Facial paralysis—Sed. LI-4, GB-20, ST-2,4,6, B-2, T-23) **(Speech difficulty**—bleed miracle points underside of tongue (½" either side of frenulum) Ton. GV-15, Sed. H-5) (Headaches bleed sun points. Sed. GB-20, Ton. K-3) (Chest congestion—Sed. P-6, VC-12, ST-40) (Weakness—Ton. VC-6, ST-36, Moxa GV-4, B-23) (Suddenly lose consciousness bleed all 12 terminal points on fingers and T-3, B-54, Sed. GV-20, GV-26) (Feels hot—Sed. LI-11, ST-43) (Stomach pain—Sed. ST-36, VC-11) (Urine reddish-yellow—Sed. B-27,28)
See PARALYSIS

STUPIDITY	(Idiocy—SP-1)
SWEATING (Hyperhidrosis)	(Spontaneous Sweating—VC-12, ST-36) add LI-4, ST-44 (Excessive persperation—LU-11, SP-15, B-17, T-10, GV-16, B-13, H-7, B-62) (Lack of persperation—L-8, SP-2, LI-4, GB-11,44, P-9, ST-43,45, LI-1,4, SI-2, LU-8) (Genital—VC-1, B-35) (Night—LU-11,4, LV-2, LI-43, B-17,40) (Continuous—B-54) (Excess—B-9, SP-16) (Special point to induce—LV-10) (Nocturnal sweating—GV-14, H-6, SI-3, B-13, VC-6,4,7, SP-6) (LU-1, VC-6, B-15, H-7, K-2) (SI-3, K-7, T-5)
SWELLING	(Of jaw—LI-1) (and pain of larynx—H-9) (Swelling under tongue—VC-23)
SYNCOPE	(GV-26, LU-11, Moxa GV-20) (LI-10, GV-20, LU-9, T-2, LV-1, H-9, P-9, SP-6, GB-43, ST-45, B-57)
TINNITUS	**K-1, GB-20, NRG, T-17,** (H-5, B-26, T-17) (LI-4,11, GB-2, T-17) (NRG bilat. LU-11, LI-1, T-1,3,5, P-6) (T-18,17,16, GB-20) add T-3,5. Two main points and one secondary point is used. (GB-20, SI-19, T-17) add T-5, GB-43, GB-34, H-3, K-1, K-6 (K-1, GB-44,20, B-10) (GB-7,8,9,18) (GV-16,14, B-62, P-7) Catarrhal—LV-4, SI-16, T-17, SI-19, LU-11, LI-4, K-3, ST-36, T-5, GB-2, T-21, GV-20,19, T-18, SI-3,5,19,16 (Otitis External—GB-1, SI-19, LI-4,11 (SI-19, LI-1) add ST-7, GV-4, GB-44, LI-1,4,5,6, T-2,3,5,8,9,10,16,17,18,19,21, SI-2,5,9,16,17,19, GB-2,3,4,10,11,43,44 (Tinnitus, headache, blurred vision nasal congettion, sore throat, slight cough, Sed. T-6, LU-7, B-20, T-17) (Sudden fright, sound in ear occur suddenly—Sed. T-21, SI-19, GB-2, T-17,3) (Congestion, phlegm in chest, buzzing in ear—Sed. ST-40, LI-4, P-6, T-3, GB-2) (Sound in ear, impaired hearing, insomnia—Sed. LV-3, GB-43,2, Ton. K-3) (Ton. VC-6, GV-20, ST-36) (Ton. B-23, VC-4, K-3) (Patient may suddenly become deaf—T-17,5, GB-41, LV-3, Sed.) ("Deficiency"—tinnitus intermittent, deafness comes gradually—K-3, B-23, GV-4, SP-6) **EAR POINTS**—INNER EAR, KIDNEY
TONGUE	(Swollen K-9) (Pain at root—VC-23, GB-20, H-5, P-7) See **MOUTH**
TONSILLITIS	See PHARYNGITIS SI-1, LU-1,11, ST-45, H-5,7, P-7, LU-2,8,10, LI-1,2,3,4,5,6,7, 11,17, T-10, SI-1,2,3, K-2,6, **acute—K-1,** GB-10,12,38,39, ST-10,11,12,38, 39,45, VC-16,20,22 **EAR POINT**—TONSIL, THROAT, DIVINE GATE, TONSIL-1,2,3,4, INTERNAL SECRETION
TRACHEITIS	(LI-4, LU-2, GV-12, P-3) (Excessive mucous cannot be expectorated—K-2, B-60, K-5, T-16, B-13) **EAR POINTS**—DIVINE GATE, TRACHEA, ASTHMA, SYMPATHETIC, ADRENAL
TRISMUS	(ST-6, LI-4) add T-17,5 (ST-6,7, T-17) add LI-1, let blood, T-1, ST-36
TUMOUR	(Breast—GB-44, ST-16, K-23,24, LI-8,10) (Mouth—LI-17) (Neck—GB-10)
URETHRITIS AND URETHRAL DISCHARGE	(B-23, VC-6,4, LV-13) add LV-8, SP-6, K-6, SP-4 (Red purulent matter—B-15,23,28, H-8, VC-4) add SP-9,6 Additional points—B-31,32,33,34,35, VC-1, K-11,9,10, SP-6, ST-25,28, VC-4,12, LV-1 **EAR POINTS**—KIDNEY, BLADDER, DIVINE GATE, URETHRA, EXT. GENITALS
URINARY INCONTINENCE	Special point **VC-6,** LV-1, H-5,8, LV-2, ST-22, SP-9,11, B-67, VC-1, B-27,28, ST-36, LU-7,9, GV-4, T-4 **EAR POINTS**—BRAIN, BLADDER
URINARY PROBLEMS	(B-23,28, VC-6,4,3) add SP-9,6, LV-1, B-24 (Tone K-3, VC-2,4, B-23,30) **EAR POINTS**—KIDNEY, BLADDER, DIVINE GATE
URINARY RETENTION	VC-6,4, K-2,11, SP-9,10, LI-9, ST-37, B-54 **EAR POINTS**—KIDNEY, BLADDER, SYMPATHETIC, EXT. GENITALS
URINARY TRACT INFECTIONS	(B-32, SP-6, ST-36, LV-8) add B-65, LI-11 **EAR POINTS,** URINARY TRACT, Corresponding Parts
VARICOSE VEINS	GV-14,12, GB-21, GV-4
VASCULAR ISCHEMIA	See PERIPHERAL VASCULAR DISEASE
VERTIGO	**LI-4, GB-20, ST-40** (Fatigue, paleness, chills—Ton. ST-36, VC-4, B-23,20) (Backache, palpitations, insomnia—Sed. **GB-20,** B-18, LV-2, Ton. K-1,3, B-23) (Anorexia—Sed. VC-12, ST-40,41, P-6) (Vertigo, tinnitus, weakness, fever—Ton. K-3, B-18,17, Sed. LV-14) (Severe pain gurgling in intestine, constipation, black stool—LV-13,14, VC-12, ST-40) (Head and eyes dizzy—GV-20, GB-20, ST-8, LV-14) add XHN-3, P-7, LV-3 (Vertigo—LU-4, ST-40, GB-20, B-16, GV-20, B-62,67,8, GV-23, GB-20, P-1, GV-19, ST-13, B-62, ST-17, B-66) (Syncope—LI-10, GV-20, LU-9, T-2, LV-1, H-9, P-9, SP-6, GB-43, ST-45, B-57) (Cerebral congestion—K-1, B-62, LI-1, LU-11, ST-36, P-7) (Meningismus—B-62, ST-13)

VOMITING	(P-6, VC-12, ST-36) add (VC-22) (ST-44, XHN-2) let blood (VC-12, LV-13, VC-17, B-20,21,23) add P-6, VC-13, ST-36, SP-6 See NAUSEA AND VOMITING
	(DO NOT TREAT ACUPUNCTURE COLLAPSE WITH THESE POINTS) **ALWAYS CHECK AND MAINTAIN AN AIRWAY**
RESUSCITATION, ASPHYXIA, CYANOSIS	**H-7, P-7, LU-9** ¼" deep or massage **K-1** 3" needle inserted at a 45° angle back towards heel **LV-3** 1" deep
WEAKNESS, COLLAPSE	**LI-15** 1" deep
ELECTRICAL SHOCK, TOXIC (LUNG AND HEART INTACT)	**K-1, P-6** **EAR POINTS**—ADRENAL, HEART OCCIPUT
SYNCOPE	**GV-26, LU-11, K-1, GV-20** Additional points: LI-10, GV-20, LU-9, T-2, LV-1, H-9, P-9, SP-6, GB-43, ST-45, B-57
APOPLEXY	**ST-36** (also reduces hypertension)
BURNS	**B-65,62,63**
COMA, OVERDOSE	**LEDUN POINT**—Between 2nd and 3rd rib in the nipple line, press with thumb heavily.
	PACEMAKER INSERTION EAR POINTS—C.P., T-8, LI 4, P-6

The preceding formulae for treatments are some of the combinations developed by Robert E. Willner, M.D., an excellent acupuncture-medicine practitioner. These and several hundred other reference points, charts and lists have been beautifully put together in the form of an Acupuncture Desk Reference, an almost essential tool in the physician's office.

In recent years, since the tremendous surge of interest in acupuncture in this country, instruments have been provided with the alleged ability to locate various acupuncture points. In our clinical experience, we have found that these machines are inconsistent and nothing more than a scientific toy. They are easily affected by variations in temperature and humidity, both ambient and on the skin, and have been known to give contradictory readings on the same patient, very much as if the acupuncture point had been moved. It is true that the skin can be stretched, but in the case of these "tobiscopes" one has the feeling that it is the imagination that does the stretching.

An exception to this idea is the French-made instrument designed for use in auriculo-therapy. It has proven itself in both research and practice to be a consistent and 90%-accurate tool in auriculo-therapy situations, far superior to the many European and American variations and copies.

Perhaps the reader is finding difficulty reconciling the lack of belief, on the part of the author, in acupuncture points and the repeated reference to this or that point in terms of the old meridian theory. It is to be remembered that learning classical acupuncture systems is a good way to start, and their historic use has never been disputed. Additionally, it provides us with somewhat universal vocabulary, transcending language barriers.

The author and Western-trained Chinese do subscribe to the following statement, which was expressed at the NIH meeting in Washington:

Quoted from
The Peking Medical Review
February 1972

> It was found that about half of the known acupunctural points are located right over various nerves and the rest are within half a centimetre of one or another nerve. From this, the conclusion was drawn that acupuncture acts in fact on the nervous system, and it is through a nerve that the stimulus produced by needling or applying a mild electric current is transmitted to a certain part or organ of the body where it effects a cure or brings about a state of analgesia.
>
> With this knowledge, additional acupunctural points have been located along the nervous system, and they are not necessarily found on any of the *ching* described hitherto. By following the nervous system, medical workers have been able to pinpoint spots which are even more effective for anaesthesia than points formerly known.

It may seem repetitious to make this statement as many times as we have, but it took this many times to get it inserted into the N.I.H. record of the meeting!

CHAPTER XI

ELECTRICAL ACUPUNCTURE "ANESTHESIA"
Report of a Series of Seven Surgical Cases

Frank Z. Warren, M.D.; Pang L. Man, M.D.; and Calvin H. Chen, M.D., M.Sc. (Med.)

Dr. Warren is former Clinical Assistant Professor of Anesthesiology, New York University Medical Center, and Director, The Sleep and Somatic Therapy Center, Postgraduate Center for Mental Health, New York; Dr. Man is Director of Research, Northville State Hospital, Northville, Michigan; Dr. Chen is Assistant Medical Superintendent, Northville State Hospital, and Adjunct Assistant Professor of Psychiatry, Wayne State University.

Reprint requests to Northville State Hospital, Northville, Michigan 47167 (Dr. Chen).

Synopsis

Between November 6, 1971 and July 1, 1972 the authors participated in seven surgical procedures in which acupuncture was used to provide the necessary "anesthesia." Except for the first case, a Chinese electrical acupuncture machine was used. The "anesthetic" and operative procedures are described, as is a neurophysiological theory (two-gate control theory) which provides a scientific explanation of the acupuncture analgesia mechanism. The differences from and advantages over conventional anesthesia are discussed.

Unconfirmed reports of operations in China with only acupuncture needles as the "anesthetic" had been circulating since

1966, but were either scoffed at as hypnosis or ignored for other reasons. The reports persisted nevertheless, and were finally corroborated by medical and lay eyewitnesses in 1971 and 1972.

Attempts to obtain specific operating room data, however, were unsuccessful. With the exception of the *JAMA* report of E. Gray Dimond,[1] no authoritative papers could be obtained. Communications to the Institute of Acupuncture Research in Peking went unanswered, and it was then revealed that the institute had closed two years earlier because of the Cultural Revolution.

The original acupuncture articles written in Chinese that reached these shores were confusing and unsatisfactory. Diplomatic sources, though polite and helpful, were not scientifically accurate. In the meantime, the roster of impressed eyewitnesses grew daily by leaps and bounds, vivified by a Chinese film of the procedures released from Peking.

Shortly before the avalanche of acupuncture information in the lay press, in the spring of 1971, the writers had been collecting a bibliography and attempting to investigate acupuncture because of incidents relative to their practice and their background. Two had been trained in China, and one had been exposed to treatment of a personal injury by acupuncture. The goals sought were, first, a scientific explanation of what they had seen, read and heard; and, second, the possibility that at some future date the Chinese results could be replicated. The authors were encouraged by early investigations on themselves and members of their families—which, in effect, served the purposes of animal experimentation—and the fact that they were able to obtain a Chinese electrical acupuncture machine and some detailed Chinese reports.

Optimally, the objective was the development of sufficient "anesthesia" to allow for surgical intervention. The basis for explaining the effects of the acupuncture "anesthesia" had been arrived at months earlier and was labeled the "two-gate control theory."[2] Briefly, this theory states that when a peripheral branch of a spinal nerve is mildly stimulated with the acupuncture needle, whether twirled or charged with a rather low voltage electric current, the A-beta fibers are stimulated. This results in the production of a steady stream of non-pain impulses which closes the first gate in the substantia gelatinosa of the spinal cord and the second (main) gate in the thalamus, thus preventing any pain sensation coming in anywhere from the C fibers from passing through these gates to reach the cortex and be felt by the patient. If a peripheral branch of a cranial nerve is stimulated, then the second gate will be closed with the same result.

Case Reports

Two of the three writers and one of their wives had undergone operations on themselves.

Case 1. On November 6, 1971, one of them (FZW) had a small scar, three centimeters in length, removed from his lumbar area in the office of a New York surgeon (MM). In this instance, two needles were placed in positions *fuai* and *ching-men* (below midtal margin of front and back, respectively). They were twirled at 100 rpm to produce the necessary surgical analgesia. Three silk skin sutures were placed; these were removed uneventfully one week later. The entire experience was satisfactory and highly educational. This case had not been reported.

Case 2. On May 13, 1972, PLM submitted himself for the excision of a piece of normal skin and subcutaneous tissue 2.5 x 1 cm. Goniz Kayi was the surgeon.

Case 3. On May 15, 1972, PLM's wife had a third molar extracted.

Cases 2 and 3 were performed at Northville State Hospital by using the Chinese electrical acupuncture machine. They were reported elsewhere.[3]

Because of these preliminary successes, four more operations were performed on volunteers, using the Chinese electrical acupuncture machine to provide the necessary surgical analgesia. The first two were performed on May 26, 1972, by Gershon Efron, a surgeon, at the Albert Einstein College of Medicine, under the supervision of Louis R. Orkin, Professor and Chairman of the Department of Anesthesiology.

The night before surgery a psychiatric examination was performed on three patient volunteers. The purpose of this was to eliminate any mental conditions such as neuroses or personality disorders that might cause any psychological trauma to the patient as the result of the use of acupuncture surgical analgesia. What also had to be guarded against were volunteers who had either psychosis, organic brain syndrome, or mental retardation, since they might not be able to report properly the presence or absence of pain. One 38-year-old female was rejected because her personality profile was definitely hysterical, while the other two were accepted and constituted cases 4 and 5 of our series. On the morning of the operation it was recognized that another pair of hands would be needed to reinforce the machines. Dr. Yoshiaki Omura was called at 7:00 a.m. and asked if he would hand-twirl a needle at L.I.4 during the operation. He performed the task admirably.

Case 4. A 40-year-old Caucasian male with a previous history of unsuccessful spinal anesthesia for a left inguinal herniorrhaphy was the first volunteer. That night the patient was given 100 mg. of sodium pentobarbital. In the morning, the usual pre-operative medications were administered before he was brought to the operating room where a solution of 500 cc. of 5% dextrose in water containing 50 mg. of meperidine was started. Needles were placed in the classical Chinese positions of *nienchu, tsusanli,* and *hoku.* The translation of these Chinese points into landmarks with which we are familiar is as follows: One needle was placed in proximity to the right supratrochlear nerve, two needles were placed in close proximity to the peroneal nerves three inches below the inferior border of the patella, and one needle was placed at the apex of the web between the first and second metacarpals of the left hand (radial nerve). The needles in *tsusanli* were connected to the machine, while the rest were twirled at approximately 100 rpm. The induction was begun at approximately 9:58 a.m., and by 10:28 a.m. neurologic skin-testing indicated sufficient analgesia had been developed that the surgical procedure could start.

A 15-cm. incision was made above and parallel to the medial 2/3 of the inguinal ligament without the discernment of pain or discomfort. The external oblique muscle was incised down to the superficial ring, and the ileo-inguinal nerve detected and placed outside the external oblique aponcurosis. The cord was mobilized and the sac dissected.

At 10:48 a.m. the surgeon began the dissection of the hernial sac itself, at which point the patient began to experience the first discomfort whenever the spermatic cord was poked or pushed by the stick-sponge forceps. The blood pressure at this point had come down from 140/90 to 112/78. The patient stated he could feel some sensation, but wished the operation to continue. He did not complain of pain, but more of a dull ache. The intensity of the current was increased in an attempt to block this. Continued testing of the operative area revealed some hypesthesia, some sensation of pressure, still no sensation of pain, but definitely some discomfort.

It was recalled that in Dimond's report the abdominal surgery patients in China were frequently uncomfortable at this stage of the operation. Accordingly, a choice of one of three ways to proceed seemed to be presented:

1. Continue with the acupuncture surgical analgesia alone, ignoring the discomfort. This was against our moral code.

2. Infiltrate with local anesthetic to get past the stripping of cord. We did not know the Chinese did this routinely.

3. Change to a general anesthetic.

Because of the lowering of blood pressure and a light diaphoresis, it was therefore decided to use the third of the alternatives. The patient was immediately put to sleep with 200 mg. of intravenous hexobarbital. By that time he had been under acupuncture analgesia exclusively for 22 minutes, and had not really objected to any part of the procedure. The meperidine-dextrose solution drip, of which 150 cc. (or 15 mg. of meperidine) had been used, was discontinued.

The operation proceeded uneventfully, and when awakened later the patient was overheard to say, "Why did you put me to sleep? I could have gone on." This was repeated in the recovery room and also downstairs in his own room to three different physicians.

Case 5. Another male patient, age 65, Caucasian, underwent a skin graft operation to cover a large ulcer of the right lower leg following osteomyelitis. This second patient of the Albert Einstein series was selected because at a previous grafting operation the spinal anesthetic apparently was unsuccessful and the patient was reported by the surgeon to have complained bitterly throughout the entire operation. The evening before, it was ascertained that his psychiatric status was satisfactory. He was premedicated with 100 mg. of pentobarbital. On the morning of the operation the usual preoperative medications were given. A meperidine drip, with 50 mg. in 500 cc. of 5% dextrose, was started.

Needles were placed in the same points as above, except for the addition of an extra needle in the left supraorbital nerve position. The needles in the supraorbital positions were electrified, while the others were twirled by hand with the assistance of Yoshiaki Omura, another member of the New York City Committee for Acupuncture Research.

The induction was begun at 12:20 p.m. Sufficient surgical analgesia had been obtained by 1:05 p.m. A Brown dermatome then proceeded to remove three split thickness grafts from the lateral anterior surface of the right thigh, each approximately 2 x 3 cm., and transplanted to the ulcerated area, which was approximately 14 x 15 cm. This area had been prepared in the usual way by debriding, and the excess granulation tissue removed by sharp dissection.

There was no question of the painfulness of the procedure without surgical analgesia, but the patient felt no pain at all, seemed quite comfortable, and was able to sip orange juice and converse throughout the entire procedure. His sensorium was entirely clear and did not at all seem impaired by any medication or the procedure itself. Eighteen sutures were placed. The entire procedure took one hour and five minutes. At the conclusion, the patient could have walked out of the operating room, but was instead helped onto a cart under his own motive power. Only 25 mg. of meperidine in the drip was used.

The following two volunteers were operated on by Ralph Cilento and Goniz Kayi, respectively, at Northville State Hospital, Northville, Michigan, on July 1, 1972:

Case 6: A 36-year-old Caucasian female had a tumor in the right deltoid area for several years. But within the last month it started to increase in size. A psychiatric evaluation showed no psychological contraindications. The night before she was premedicated with 400 mg. of meprobamate. On the morning of the operation she was given no medication. She was brought to the operating room, where her blood pressure was found to be 140/85, pulse 90 per minute, and the remaining physical signs essentially negative.

A 500-cc. drip of 5% dextrose in water, mixed with 60 mg. of meperidine, was started. Acupuncture needles were then placed above the eyebrows in the *yang pai* position (supraorbital nerve) and in the anterior aspect of ear lobule in the *yang tai* position (greater auricular nerve). Each pair of needles was connected to the machine.

Induction of surgical analgesia was begun at 10:00 a.m., and achieved in 30 minutes. At 10:30 a.m. a skin incision about 3 cm. long was made without evidence of pain. The subcutaneous tissue was dissected, the lipoma, 2 x 2 cm. in diameter, was removed, and eight black silk sutures were placed. Closure was completed at 10:51 a.m. The total operating time was 21 minutes. One hundred fifty cc. of the intravenous solution (or 18 mg. of meperidine) was used. The patient was able to walk out of the operating room.

Case 7. A Caucasian female, age 56, complaining of a tumor in the left side of the posterior neck overlying the trapezius, approximately 3 x 3 cm. in diameter, had volunteered for the operation. Her psychiatric examination was essentially normal. The night before surgery she was given 5 mg. of diazepam. In the morning she was brought to the operating room and placed on the operating table on her right side. A mixture of 500 cc. of 5% dextrose in water and 60 mg. of meperidine was started intravenously.

Needles were placed in the same positions and connected to the machines as in case 6. Induction began at 11:15 a.m., and at 11:45 a.m. sufficient analgesia had developed to begin the operation. At 11:46 a.m. a 4-cm. skin incision was made and the underlying fatty tissue was exposed. The lipoma, rather deep seated, was dissected with scissors from the overlying skin and subcutaneous tissue and removed with no evidence of pain. Six interrupted No. 40 silk sutures were placed. The procedure took approximately 25 minutes. Again 150 cc. of the intravenous fluid (or 18 mg. of meperidine) was used.

These observations have not been previously published. It was decided to withhold them for inclusion in this book rather than have them published in a magazine.

Comment

In our opinion, the seven operations described in this paper were all successful, and the two-gate control theory serves to explain the mechanism of acupuncture "anesthesia" in a scientific way based on modern neuroanatomy and neurophysiology. What we must emphasize to the readers at this point is the difference between classical Chinese acupuncture and acupuncture "anesthesia." Classical acupuncture, through years of usage, had accumulated a great many notions tinged with mysticism and occultism. On the other hand, "modern" acupuncture was fairly recent, starting with the constant twirling and then the electrifying of the needle which made it possible to provide "anesthesia" for surgical operations. Another point which needs to be clarified is that the "anesthesia" produced by acupuncture differs noticeably from conventional anesthesia; the former blocks only pain sensation, while the latter blocks all sensations, including nonpainful ones. Thus it is more accurate to call the "anesthesia" produced by the modern acupuncture technique "surgical analgesia." It was only with this pain-blocking aspect of acupuncture that the writers' investigations were concerned.

Acupuncture surgical analgesia has a number of advantages: 1. It is simple, safe, economical, and relatively easy to administer. 2. It may be used in patients in whom the conventional general or local anesthesia is risky or contraindicated. 3. Because the patient is conscious, it is particularly useful in operations in which the patient's cooperation is helpful or required. 4. The fact that the needles may be placed anywhere in the body to produce surgical analgesia anywhere else (without regard to the traditional acupuncture points) makes it possible to avoid the necessity of the anesthesiologist and the surgeon occupying the same area. 5. The electrical acupuncture machine is to be preferred because it obviates the need for assistants to crowd around the operating field to do the very fatiguing and boring job of twirling the needles.

Three other observations are of interest. First, all patients except case 4 did not have any postoperative pain. So far we are not yet able to offer an explanation. Second, case 6 stated that she thought the incision was circular instead of linear. It is possible that there was some involvement of the cerebral cortex causing a perception distortion. Third, in cases 6 and 7 the voltage used in the ear lobule position was several times higher than that used in the supraorbital position. This might be due to the fact that the peripheral nerves in the former are much smaller.

Finally we wish to state that from our experiences so far, electrical acupuncture surgical analgesia is worthy of further intensive and extensive investigation.

REFERENCES

1. Dimond, E.G.: Acupuncture anesthesia, Western medicine and Chinese traditional medicine. JAMA, 218:1558-1563, 1971.
2. Man P.L., Chen C.H.: The mechanism of acupuncture "anesthesia": the two-gate control theory. Dis Nerv Syst. In press.
3. Man P.L., Chen C.H.: Acupuncture "anesthesia": a new theory and clinical study. Cur Ther Res 14:390-394, 1972.

CHAPTER XII

ACUPUNCTURE AND THE LAW

William H. L. Dornette, M.D., J.D.

Director of Education and Research, Division of Anesthesiology, Cleveland Clinic, Cleveland, Ohio; Member of the Ohio Bar.

Reprinted with permission from the Journal of Legal Medicine, Vol. 2 (No. 2, March/April), 1974. Data have been brought up to date and are current as of April 1, 1975.

The recent events that have led to the introduction of acupuncture into American professional practice are well known. While new to most physicians, dentists, and other scientists, acupuncture is of course thousands of years old in discovery and application. The origins of acupuncture and Oriental explanations of its mode of action stir the fantasy of the Western physician.

These explanations defy Western science, rooted as they are in the magic and mysticism of the East. For this reason, plus the seemingly miraculous cures often wrought by acupuncture, organized medicine in America has tended to reject acupuncture as a viable, valid therapeutic modality, or at least to take an overly cautious view of it.

Thus, while the curiosity of the physician may result only in that—curiosity but no action—the laymen's curiosity may result in positive action. If he is suffering from an illness which he *believes* will, or may, be helped by acupuncture, he is going to *actively* seek help. This imbalance between needed and available services has already created significant problems. First, there has been a proliferation of acupuncture treatment "centers" in some of the larger cities, staffed principally by foreign-trained acupuncturists who have no professional degree and whose command of the English language leaves much to be desired. Additionally, there has been a lag in the development and application of acupuncture by members of the profession as a whole.

Additionally, foreign-trained acupuncturists, with or without professional degrees, have come to this country to utilize, or attempt to utilize, acupuncture in various areas, notably in larger cities. The Department of Labor has had numerous requests for immigrant visas from individuals claiming to be acupuncturists but not licensed in any branch of the healing arts in their own country.

Fortunately for the general health and well-being of the American public, the Food and Drug Administration (FDA) and the majority of the healing-arts licensing boards have taken formal positions on the use of acupuncture. This chapter reviews the current legal status of these positions. The acupuncture enthusiast who wonders about the diversity of positions taken by the healing arts boards in the various states or questions the strong position of the FDA should review the source of the authority of these various agencies.

The authority of the FDA rests in the public laws, enacted by the Congress, which created the agency and gave it its powers over drugs and devices. The power of the Congress to enact this legislation rests in the United States Constitution. This power to create the FDA and give it its own powers is derived from two specific sections of the Constitution. The Preamble states that the Constitution is established to promote the general welfare. Article 1, §1, establishes the legislative power of the Congress; §8, Clause 3, states in part: ". . . the Congress shall have the power . . . to regulate commerce . . . among the several States. . . ."

Thus the Congress clearly has the power to enact legislation that regulates commerce in furtherance of the general welfare. No one has made serious efforts to challenge the fundamental purpose of the FDA, namely, to promote the health and general welfare of the people of the United States by regulating drugs and medical devices sold in interstate commerce.

In furtherance of its responsibilities to the American public, the FDA called a meeting of experts and other interested parties to discuss the possible regulation of acupuncture. The meeting was held in Washington, D.C., on September 22, 1972. Those attending the meeting included representatives of the American Medical

Association, American Society of Anesthesiologists, the Federation of State Medical Boards, the National Institutes of Health, certain states, and the city of New York. Individual medical practitioners and the Medical Devices Advisory Committee of the FDA also attended. Physicians thus were well represented. The *unanimous* consensus of those attending this meeting was that the use of acupuncture constitutes an experimental procedure and that the equipment used—needles and electrical generators for stimulation—are experimental devices.

The thrust of the resulting regulation is simple and straightforward. It applies to devices sold in interstate commerce, whether they are new or already in general use, as long as the application is experimental. (Thus, a nerve stimulator, an accepted device manufactured to test viability and response of nerve trunks and in use long before September 1971, would constitute an "experimental device" if used for acupuncture.) The device must be labeled as being experimental. Labeling suggested by the FDA states: "Caution: Experimental device limited to investigational use by or under the direct supervision of a licensed physician or dental practitioner. This device should be used only with informed consent under conditions designed to protect the patient as a research subject, where the scientific protocol for investigation has been reviewed and approved by an appropriate institutional review committee and where conditions for safe use are in accordance with state law."

In the case of acupuncture needles, the packaging must be so labeled. Finally, the informed consent of the patient (as discussed below) must be obtained.

In theory, the acupuncturist could circumvent this regulation by manufacturing his own needles and manipulating them digitally. Or, if he has a knowledge of electronics or access to someone who has, he could build his own electrical stimulator or have it built for him. While this course of action might not be violating the letter of the law, it certainly would be at odds with the spirit of this regulation. The best and safest course for all acupuncture practitioners to take would be to abide by the FDA regulations. If an acupuncturist built his own device or had it built for him, from a form or from scratch, he should affix a label to it containing the cautionary statement of the FDA. And he should *always* obtain the informed consent of each of his patients.

The practice of the healing arts, like the practice of law and other professions, is a privilege granted by the state on demonstration of the necessary expertise by licensure or bar examination.

This restriction on professional practice is a function of the government of each individual state. The power to restrict professional practice flows to each licensing board from the United States Constitution, through the respective state constitutions and legislatures. While the powers of the federal government under the Constitution are broad when a national or interstate problem is involved, they are very limited by the Bill of Rights to these two specific areas. The states and the people retain certain broad powers under Article X: "The powers not delegated to the United States by the Constitution, nor prohibited by it to the States, are reserved to the States respectively, or to the people." Among these powers is the one to promote the health and well-being of the citizens of the individual states. These powers, further enumerated in the constitution of each state, enable the respective legislatures to enact laws creating healing-arts licensing boards and empowering them to act.

How each board acts on a specific question will depend on a variety of factors. But because of the press of business that regularly comes before a board and the fact that board members generally are engaged in the full-time practice of their profession, it is not likely that a given board will act on a question that has not been presented to it. It is to be expected, therefore, that some boards may not have adopted a position.

In the latter part of August 1973, I commenced a mail survey of the positions of all state (initially, medical) licensing boards. Some six months, 123 letters, and 36 follow-up long distance telephone calls later, the study was completed; data were obtained from all 51 dental, and the 21 separate osteopathic, licensing boards. (All jurisdictions have combined medical-osteopathic licensing boards except: Arizona, Arkansas, California, Connecticut, Florida, Hawaii, Louisiana, Maine, Michigan, Montana, Nevada, New Mexico, North Carolina, Oklahoma, Pennsylvania, Rhode Island, Tennessee, Utah, Vermont, Washington, and West Virginia.) These data were published in the March-April 1974 issue of the *Journal of Legal Medicine*. In January of 1975 I repeated the process to make the information current.

A compilation of these data (Tables 1 and 2) reveals some diversity of positions across the country. This diversity, which may confuse the healing arts practitioner, is understandable. The powers retained by the states to regulate the healing arts rest in large measure solely within each state. The licensing board thus would be expected to adopt regulations that would meet the specific problems encountered or expected to be encountered within that state, and none other. The rights of states to regulate healing-arts practice in this manner is a healthy one, commensurate with the best traditions of the republic.

The legalistic processes by which the individual licensing boards have adopted their positions are interesting. Some obtained an opinion from the attorney general of the state. Others have been able to resort to the statutory definition of the practice of their particular branch of the healing arts, and have attempted to fit acupuncture into that definition. In some, the legislature has enacted a statute. In others, a special commission was convened to draft a position paper which was subsequently adopted by the respective healing-arts licensing board.

Generally, what constitutes professional practice is defined in the state statute that regulates it. The Wisconsin and Oregon dental examining boards achieved opposite results by this method. The Oregon board reasoned that since acupuncture is used for the treatment of pain, both operative and pathological, it constitutes the practice of dentistry, since the dental practitioner is permitted by statute to use agents and techniques to allay pain. The Wisconsin statute provides that a dentist licensed in the state may perform any procedure taught in an accredited dental school within the state. Since acupuncture is not a part of the curriculum of either dental school in Wisconsin, the Wisconsin Board of Dental Examiners initially held that acupuncture could not be practiced legally in that state. This position has been changed, however (see Table 2).

Some practitioners may be at a loss to understand why a number of licensing boards have taken no position on acupuncture whatsoever. To the acupuncture enthusiast, this lack of any position may seem incongruous and suggest laziness or "fence riding." It can be explained readily because of the newness (to Western medicine) of the technique and the fact that judicial and quasi-judicial bodies are reticent to act upon an issue that has not yet been formally presented to them. Thus, if no practitioner in a given jurisdiction has elected to use the technique, a state licensing board will have no pressing need to take a position.

Physicians and dentists are referred to Tables 1 and 2, respectively, for the positions taken by the licensing board in their state. Some of these positions will be discussed, however, because of their restrictive nature.

Twenty-one of the states (e.g., Arizona, Arkansas, California) have separate medical and osteopathic licensing boards. The other 30 jurisdictions (e.g., Alabama, Alaska, Colorado) have combined boards. The large majority of these boards have adopted the position that acupuncture is the practice of medicine or osteopathy. Only one state, Indiana, forbids the use of acupuncture by licensed physicians. The medical board in Indiana is awaiting the outcome of research being conducted at the University of Indiana.

In 15 states, the medical boards have taken the position that acupuncture is experimental, and various research guidelines must be followed, including obtaining the informed consent of the patient. These states include Alabama, Arizona, Colorado, Delaware, Georgia, Kansas, Louisiana, Maryland, Nebraska, New York, Oklahoma, Pennsylvania, Rhode Island, Tennessee, and Utah. The Ohio Board has adopted the position of the FDA, namely, that the equipment used for acupuncture is experimental. As such, it must be properly labeled, and the patient must be informed of its experimental nature.

The recent amendments of the Food and Drug Laws require that informed consent be obtained from the subject of research. The FDA's statement in the *Federal Register* of March 9, 1973[1] reiterates the need for informed consent when employing acupuncture equipment. The medical boards in Arizona, Delaware, Indiana, New York, Ohio, Pennsylvania, Tennessee, and Utah require that this informed consent be documented. While I am in general opposed to the use of *forms* to document *informed* consent (in contrast to consent to the treatment itself), I do believe that such a form can be used when dealing with acupuncture. A recommended form appears with this chapter. Before asking the patient to sign this form, the acupuncturist must explain to the patient the nature of the procedure, expected results, and likely complications, as compared to the same aspects of alternative forms of treatment or none at all. That is, the acupuncturist must give the patient an understanding of the risk/benefit ratio.

At least five states have adopted acupuncture legislation. Alaska and Arizona allow physician's assistants to become licensed to perform acupuncture, provided certain qualifications are met. Licensing of non-physician acupuncturists can be accomplished in Hawaii, Nebraska, and Nevada, the latter through a special Board of Chinese Medicine.[2]

Special training of the physician who desires to practice acupuncture is required in California, Connecticut, Delaware, Montana, Nevada, New York, and Ohio.

The medical boards in eleven jurisdictions do permit the use of acupuncture by a non-physician if working under the direct supervision of a licensed practitioner. These jurisdictions are Alaska, Arizona, California (only in a medical school), the District of Columbia, Florida, Maine, Massachusetts, New York, Oregon, Tennessee, and Texas. Non-licensed assistants are specifically excluded in Oklahoma.

While the medical and osteopathic boards in Vermont and Washington and the osteopathic board in Connecticut have taken no position on acupuncture, it is advisable for any physician desiring to practice acupuncture in one of these states to be duly licensed.

Penalties that might accrue to the practitioner who violates a provision of the licensing board in his jurisdiction would depend upon the nature of the violation. All state statutes provide that the unlicensed practice of medicine, osteopathy, or dentistry is a felony punishable by imprisonment or fine, or both. Aiding and abetting unlicensed professional practice is also a crime. Thus, the acupuncturist must be licensed in all jurisdictions except those eleven that specifically allow an acupuncturist to function under the direct supervision of a licensed physician.

Of the dental licensing boards, 26 have not adopted positions on acupuncture as of April 1, 1975. The board in one state—Vermont—is still considering the adoption of a position.

Special training of the acupuncturist is required in Delaware, Montana, New York, Ohio, and Wisconsin. Special licensure is required in Hawaii. A "hospital setting" is required in the District of Columbia. Acupuncture is considered to be an experimental procedure, with appropriate research guidelines and safeguards to be followed, and informed consent obtained, in Delaware, New Jersey, New York, Pennsylvania, Rhode Island, and South Dakota ("a controlled scientific situation"). The Ohio Board considers the equipment to be experimental and requires that the dental practitioner follow FDA guidelines.

Dental practitioners are not permitted to use acupuncture in Michigan, Nebraska, Rhode Island, Texas, Utah, and Wisconsin.

Dentists practicing in one of the 26 states whose dental boards have not adopted a position on acupuncture should proceed with caution. The medical board's position may specifically preclude non-physicians from using acupuncture.

Physicians and dentists are all aware of the malpractice implications of the practice of medicine at the present time. The possibility that acupuncture will be associated with iatrogenic complications may seem remote—it probably is. Nevertheless, breakage of a needle, the production of a pneumothorax or other trauma, or the transmission of hepatitis is possible. The common-law proof of negligence, which unfortunately seems to be applied to the practice of Western medicine with increasing frequency, would be identical in the case of negligently administered acupuncture therapy. Furthermore, a physician or dentist will always be held vicariously liable for the negligence of a non-licensed acupuncturist working under his supervision.

Thus, it is obvious that the practitioner must be assured of coverage by his professional liability insurance carrier for any problems arising from the use of acupuncture. Because of the newness of the technique, it is possible that many carriers have not considered it in their rate making. Because the technique, on its face, does not appear to be based on scientific principles, some carriers may be reticent to offer coverage. At least one carrier has refused to cover not only the practitioner himself but physicians who refer cases to him! Other carriers may require a special Acupuncture Exclusion Endorsement. One such endorsement reads:

> It is hereby agreed and understood that this insurance does not apply to the use of the procedure known as acupuncture performed by/or at the direction of/or with the permission of/or under the control of Named Insured unless provided for by an endorsement hereto, signed by a Company Officer, with the appropriate additional deposit PAID.
>
> All other terms and conditions of this policy remain unchanged.

Having observed and administered acupuncture, I sincerely believe that the use of this technique by a duly licensed practitioner, who has training in acupuncture and a thorough knowledge of anatomy, poses no more, and probably far less, risk to the patient than many other therapeutic modalities. Thus, there should be no increase in exposure to alleged malpractice, and hence no increased cost of professional liability insurance. Obviously, the physician or dentist must adhere to any limitations imposed by his licensing board. The guidelines of the FDA also should be followed. While it may be neither negligence nor illegal practice to deviate from these recommendations, a failure to follow them might create an inference of negligence in the eyes of lay jurors should a complication and subsequent litigation ensue.

As noted above, the medical licensing boards in 2 states, the separate osteopathic boards in 3 states, and the dental boards in 26 states have not adopted a position on acupuncture as of the time of this writing. While this failure to act is understandable, it is unfortunate from several standpoints. First, it does not discourage the practice of acupuncture by non-licensed individuals, and may even result in such individuals entering this country to practice in those states. To quote from a position statement of the Minnesota State Board of Medical Examiners: "Acupuncture is here and time is of the essence to prevent it from being taken over by unqualified persons and irregular cultists."[3] Second, it may deter the legitimate practice of acupuncture by professionals who are duly licensed. For example, assume that a dental practitioner desires to use acupuncture analgesia, proven to be a safe and satisfactory substitute for local anesthesia in dentistry. If he practices in a state in which the dental board has taken no position but the medical board has held acupuncture to be the practice of medicine, it could be construed to be unlawful for the dentist to use acupuncture.

It is my firm conviction that each healing-arts licensing board in every state should adopt a position on acupuncture. If the board agrees that acupuncture should be permitted within the jurisdiction, its application should be limited to duly licensed practitioners. Whether the practitioner may employ a non-licensed assistant and whether research limitations are to be imposed would be up to the discretion of each individual board.

For those licensed practitioners who desire to employ acupuncture, but who are deterred by present regulations in their jurisdiction, a word of hope may be offered. As the value of acupuncture is developed, through properly conducted research, so too will the law develop. A noted jurist, Benjamin Cardozo, wrote in 1924: "Existing legal rules and principles can give us our present location, our bearings, our latitude and longitude. The inn that shelters for the night is not the journey's end. The law, like the traveler, must be ready for the morrow. It must have the principle of growth."[4]

Clearly, the law does grow. And, in the case of acupuncture as in countless other medical areas, it will grow, commensurate with the needs of the profession and our patients.

REFERENCES

1. 38 Fed. Reg. 6419 (Mar. 9, 1973).
2. Nev. Rev. Stats. tit. 54 §2-24.
3. Minn. State Bd. of Medical Examiners: News Release, Nov. 18, 1973.
4. Cardozo, B.N., Growth of the Law 20 (1924).

Informed Consent to Acupuncture

1. I will hereby agree to the performance of acupuncture on:

   ____
   (Insert myself or name of patient)

   for the purpose of treating ________________________
   (Insert diagnosis)

   or for the performance of acupuncture analgesia.

2. I understand that the acupuncture will be performed by, or

   under the direct supervision of ____________________,
   (Insert name and degree of practitioner)

   a physician / dentist licensed to practice in the state of ____________.

3. I further understand that acupuncture is an experimental procedure at the present time and that no guarantee can be or is made as to the success of this form of therapy. Alternative forms of therapy, and the likelihood of their success in the treatment of my condition, have been explained to me..

________________ ____________________________
Witness — Signature of patient, next of kin or legal guardian

________________ ____________________________
Date — Relationship to patient (if patient is unable to sign form)

POSITIONS ON ACUPUNCTURE OF STATE HEALING ARTS LICENSING BOARDS

compiled by
William H. L. Dornette, M.D., J.D.

Note: The following tables give the positions on acupuncture of each state licensing board for the healing arts. Table 1 covers the medical and osteopathic boards, Table 2 the dental boards. The practitioner who plans to use acupuncture must be familiar with and abide by the position of his respective board. In some cases (e.g., Georgia, New York) the requirements are detailed and strict. Special licensure may be required in other states (e.g., Hawaii, Nevada). Table 3 summarizes the position of the Federal Food and Drug Administration.

These data are current as of April 1, 1975. Positions do change, however. Neither the author who researched these positions nor the National Acupuncture Research Society is responsible for the absolute accuracy of these data. THE PROFESSIONAL WHO DESIRES TO EMPLOY ACUPUNCTURE AND WHO HAS ANY DOUBTS ABOUT THE POSITION OF HIS OWN LICENSING BOARD SHOULD CONTACT THAT BOARD. Such is especially the case in Georgia, Hawaii, Montana, Nevada and New York.

Table 1—Positions of State Medical and Osteopathic Licensing Boards

(Numbers refer to Notes at end of Tables)

	Practice of medicine or osteopathy; must be licensed	Training in acupuncture required	May be performed by non-licensee if under direct supervision of license holder	Experimental	May be performed only in a hospital setting	Informed consent required	Other (see notes at end of table)
Alabama	•			•		•	
Alaska	•		1				
Arizona Medical	•		•2	•	•		3
Osteopathic	•						
Arkansas Medical	•						
Osteopathic	•						

California Medical	●		4			
Osteopathic	●	●				
Colorado	●			5		
Connecticut Medical	●	●				
Osteopathic						no position
Delaware	●	●		●	●	6
District of Columbia			7			
Florida Medical	●		●			
Osteopathic	●		●			
Georgia	●			●	●	8
Hawaii Medical	●9					
Osteopathic	●9					

	Practice of medicine or osteopathy; must be licensed	Training in acupuncture required	May be performed by non-licensee if under direct supervision of license holder	Experimental	May be performed only in a hospital setting	Informed consent required	Other (see notes at end of table)
Idaho	•						
Illinois	•						
Indiana							10
Iowa	•						
Kansas	•			11			
Kentucky	•						
Louisiana Medical	•						12
Osteopathic	•						12
Maine Medical	•		•				
Osteopathic	•						

Maryland	•					13
Massachusetts	•		14			
Michigan Medical	•					15
Osteopathic						16
Minnesota	•					17
Mississippi	•			•		18
Missouri	•					
Montana Medical		•				19
Osteopathic		•				19
Nebraska	•			•	•	20
Nevada Medical	•	•				21
Osteopathic	•	•				21
New Hampshire	•					

	Practice of medicine or osteopathy; must be licensed	Training in acupuncture required	May be performed by non-licensee if under direct supervision of license holder	Experimental	May be performed only in a hospital setting	Informed consent required	Other (see notes at end of table)
New Jersey	•						
New Mexico Medical	•						
Osteopathic							22
New York	•	•		•		•	23
North Carolina Medical	•						
Osteopathic	•						
North Dakota	•24						
Ohio	•	•		•		•	25
Oklahoma Medical	•		26	•	•		

Osteopathic	•					
Oregon	•	•				
Pennsylvania Medical	•		•	•		
Osteopathic			•			27
Rhode Island Medical	•					
Osteopathic	•					
South Carolina	•	•28				
South Dakota	•					29
Tennessee Medical	•	•	•	•	•	
Osteopathic	•	•				
Texas	•		•			30
Utah Medical	•		•	•	•	

	Practice of medicine or osteopathy; must be licensed	Training in acupuncture required	May be performed by non-licensee if under direct supervision of license holder	Experimental	May be performed only in a hospital setting	Informed consent required	Other (see notes at end of table)
Osteopathic	•			•	•	•	
Vermont Medical							no position
Osteopathic							no position
Virginia	•			•			31
Washington Medical							no position
Osteopathic							no position
West Virginia Medical	•						
Osteopathic	•						
Wisconsin	•						
Wyoming	•						

NOTES TO TABLE 1

1. Acupuncture may be performed by duly licensed physician's assistant who meets "those requirements of experience or education in the practice of acupuncture as may be required by the board." Alaska Stats. §08.64.207.

2. "Non-physician acupuncturists may be registered as physician's assistants provided they meet established qualifications and requirements for registration" and are duly trained in acupuncture in Arizona.

3. "Any physician licensed by the Board and prescribing acupuncture shall submit quarterly reports consisting of the diagnosis, treatment and patient response to the Board of Medical Examiners or to a committee designated by the Board. The usual and legal confidentiality of patient medical records shall be maintained" in the state of Arizona.

4. If the acupuncturist is not licensed, he can only practice in a California medical school under the direct supervision of a licensed practitioner.

5. Acupuncture "should be performed" in a research environment in Colorado.

6. Research proposal must be submitted to and permit obtained from special committee of Delaware Medical Council.

7. "Acupuncture must be performed under the direct and immediate supervision of a licensed physician" in the District of Columbia.

8. FDA guidelines shall be followed; practitioners shall submit scientific protocol for investigation to institutional review committee; practitioner shall also submit application to Board of Medical Examiners (Rules of Composite Georgia State Board of Medical Examiners, Chap. 360-6, Acupuncture, 12/10/74).

9. Hawaii enacted a statute which became effective June 12, 1974. It provides for the establishment of an acupuncture board of examiners. On meeting the qualifications and passing an examination, a practitioner may be licensed to use acupuncture.

10. Until research report emanates from Indiana University, no acupuncture is to be performed by others in the state.

11. If a physician desires to conduct research on acupuncture, he shall apply to the Kansas Board of Healing Arts for a permit.

12. Acupuncture "shall be conducted only under the supervision and sponsorship of any one of the three medical schools in Louisiana for the purpose of research and study of the possible uses of acupuncture, and only under the direct supervision and responsibility of a medically licensed practitioner in Louisiana who is a member of the school staff."

13. The Maryland Board is in the process of drafting regulations for the licensure of acupuncturists.

14. Acupuncture is the practice of medicine and may be performed only 1) by a physician fully registered in the Commonwealth of Massachusetts, or 2) by an acupuncturist in the employ of this physician after examination

of the patient by this physician, consultation of this physician with the acupuncturist, and written authorization by this physician. This physician retains full legal responsibility for the competence of the acupuncturist, for the acupuncture and any and all consequences thereof.

15. The Michigan Board of Registration in Medicine regards "the practice of acupuncture as a treatment method requiring further investigation. Such investigation should be carried out only in medical centers, hospitals or other institutions capable of pursuing human medical research and having suitable committees who provide the necessary peer review of protocols and appropriate monitoring of the studies."

16. Procedure is experimental; the Michigan Osteopathic Board does not condone its use at present.

17. In Minnesota the practitioner "must be qualified" in the technique.

18. "Acupuncture may be performed in the State of Mississippi only by a physician licensed to practice medicine and surgery or a dentist licensed to practice dentistry in this state. It shall be conducted only under the supervision and sponsorship of the University of Mississippi School of Medicine or School of Dentistry, Jackson, Mississippi for the purpose of research and study of the possible uses of acupuncture, and only under the direct supervision and responsibility of a medically licensed practitioner or legally licensed dentist in Mississippi who is a member of the school staff."

19. A practitioner duly licensed to practice medicine may utilize acupuncture in Montana provided that he has taken a course in the subject and has passed an examination as provided in the Revised Code on Montana, §66-3401 et seq. (effective 7/1/74).

20. Acupuncture in Nebraska "is presently experimental and restricted to duly licensed physicians engaged in research at medical schools after having acquired the permission of the 'board,' medical school authorities, and the review of the research by a peer committee."

21. Nevada has a Board of Chinese Medicine which offers licensure upon examination to qualified non-physician acupuncturists. Physicians otherwise duly licensed may practice acupuncture without licensing by the Board of Chinese Medicine, unless they desire to hold themselves out to the public as acupuncturists.

22. New Mexico Osteopathic Board "favors the continued study and evaluation of acupuncture."

23. Must be licensed and registered as a physician in the state; must present evidence satisfactory to the Department of Registration of having attained at least 50 hours of didactic instruction and clinical demonstrations on basic techniques of acupuncture and at least 50 hours of didactic and clinical instruction in advanced techniques; may be administered only within provisions of a research protocol submitted to an institutional review committee and to the Department of Registration; informed consent of patients required.

24. Pending receipt of opinion from attorney general of North Dakota.

25. In Ohio, acupuncture equipment is experimental; FDA guidelines (see Federal Register 38:6419—March 9, 1973) shall be followed; practitioner must have "completed a course of study in acupuncture under the administration of an approved college of medicine, college of osteopathy or college of podiatry."

26. Non-licensed acupuncturists specifically excluded in Oklahoma.

27. Acupuncture is experimental, and opinion of the Pennsylvania Osteopathic Board is reserved until the efficacy of this technique has been fully documented.

28. In South Carolina, acupuncture may be performed under the direct supervision of a licensed physician or dentist in a facility approved by the Department of Health and Environmental Control.

29. In South Dakota, "acupuncture shall be used only in a controlled scientific situation until such time as all future indications and contraindications for its use can be established."

30. Safety of acupuncture has not yet been established in the opinion of the Texas Board.

31. Regulations on the practice of acupuncture may be promulgated by the Virginia Board of Medicine.

Table 2—Positions of State Dental Licensing Boards

	No Position	Position
Alabama		Acupuncture is the practice of dentistry; can be performed only by a licensed practitioner as an experimental procedure; research guidelines must be followed.
Alaska		Must be licensed to practice dentistry.
Arizona	•	
Arkansas	•	
California	•	
Colorado	•	
Connecticut		Agree with 1973 position of A.D.A. Council on Research: "the premature use of acupuncture in dental procedures is to be discouraged until its potential hazards are better known and a more scientific basis for its use is clearly established."
Delaware		Procedure is experimental; informed consent is required; acupuncturist must be trained; research proposal must be submitted to and permission obtained from special committee (same position as the Medical Council of Delaware).
District of Columbia		Licensed dentist can perform acupuncture in hospital setting without a licensed physician being present; acupuncture needs further investi-

		gation; it is experimental, and informed consent is required.
Florida	•	
Georgia	•	
Hawaii		A statute which became effective June 12, 1974, provides for the establishment of an acupuncture Board of Examiners. On meeting the qualifications and passing an examination, a practitioner may be licensed to use acupuncture.
Idaho	•	
Illinois	•	
Indiana	•	
Iowa	•	
Kansas		On July 8, 1972, the Kansas State Board of Healing Arts took the position ". . . that acupuncture is not an accepted form of therapy to be applied by any branch of the healing arts." The Board does allow a practitioner to employ acupuncture as an experimental procedure after application to the Board.
Kentucky	•	
Louisiana	•	
Maine	•	
Maryland	•	
Massachusetts	•	Board of Dental Examiners has endorsed Massachusetts House Bill 1685.

	No Position	Position
Michigan		By opinion from Attorney General's office, acupuncture is not the practice of dentistry, and cannot be used lawfully by dental practitioners.
Minnesota	•	
Mississippi	•	
Missouri	•	
Montana		Practitioner duly licensed to practice dentistry may practice acupuncture only after he has taken a course in the subject and passed an examination as provided in Revised Code of Montana, §66-3401 et seq. (effective 7/1/74).
Nebraska		Acupuncture is practice of medicine only—dentists cannot use technique.
Nevada	•	
New Hampshire	•	
New Jersey		Experimental procedure; "research may be conducted only by qualified investigators at an approved institution."
New Mexico		No position at time material goes to press; regulations adopted at meeting held May 7, 1975.
New York		Must be licensed and registered as a dentist in the state; must present evidence satisfactory to the Department of Registration of having attained at least 50 hours of didactic instruction

		and clinical demonstrations on basic techniques of acupuncture and at least 50 hours of didactic and clinical instruction in advanced techniques; may be administered only within provisions of a research protocol submitted to an institutional review committee and to the Department of Registration; informed consent of patients required.
North Carolina		Should be performed only by qualified physicians and dentists.
North Dakota	•	
Ohio		The acupuncturist must be trained; the equipment used is experimental; informed consent of the patient is required; FDA guidelines for experimental devices must be followed; special training is required (same position as the Board of Medical Examiners).
Oklahoma	•	
Oregon		Acupuncture is the practice of dentistry and may be performed by practitioners licensed in the state.
Pennsylvania		Acupuncture is limited to licensed professionals, including dentists.
Rhode Island		Cannot be utilized by dentists; limited by 1974 statute to licensed physicians.
South Carolina		"Acupuncture may be performed by or under the direct supervision of a licensed dentist in a facility approved by the Department of Health and Environmental Control."

	No Position	Position
South Dakota		Acupuncture is the practice of dentistry; "a controlled scientific situation" is required (same position as the Board of Medical Examiners).
Tennessee	•	
Texas		Acupuncture is not currently recognized as an accepted therapeutic modality for use by dental practitioners.
Utah		Acupuncture is the practice of medicine or osteopathy; dental practitioners cannot use the technique.
Vermont	•	The subject is still under consideration.
Virginia		Acupuncture is the practice of dentistry; dental licensure is required (same position as the Board of Medical Examiners).
Washington	•	
West Virginia	•	
Wisconsin		Must be licensed; "thorough training and indoctrination" in acupuncture required.
Wyoming	•	

TABLE 3

SUMMARY OF POSITION ON ACUPUNCTURE OF FOOD AND DRUG ADMINISTRATION

The equipment is experimental.

Stimulators must be labeled with an experimental device notice.

Study must be conducted under the auspices and with the consent of an institutional research committee.

Informed consent of subject must be obtained and documented.

reference: 38 Federal Register 6419 (March 9, 1973)

CHAPTER XIII

MEDICAL-LEGAL ASPECTS, WEST

Leonard A. Worthington, LL.B., J.D.

The history of medical and legal literature reflects the attempt of society to protect itself against ignorant and unethical practitioners whose actions are injurious to the general public. This method of protection has assumed many facets of regulatory procedures, varying from national and state supervision to that which has been placed exclusively under the control of the universities in some countries.

The art of acupuncture involves the penetration of the flesh by needles, and therefore would come within the control and regulation of the duly constituted licensing body.

The field of medicine is initially divided into that of the physician and that of the surgeon, the latter's range of services including any act which involves the penetration of the flesh with instrumentation, however slight. It would follow, therefore, that the subject of acupuncture falls most logically within the field of surgery, whether its function is anesthetic, analgesic, or surgical in character, as this term is commonly understood.

As to responsibility of the medical profession concerning this matter, as the only body authorized by law to engage in surgery, it is obvious that unless it completes a thorough investigation in this field, it will allow a gap in the healing art which would leave the door open for invasion by other groups to assert a right of action as coming within their jurisdiction by default on the part of the duly constituted authority to act under its statutory obligation to do so.

Since this activity is included within the scope of the practice of medicine or surgery, a direct and specific duty is imposed upon the medical profession to assume the highest degree of responsibility in its efforts to exhaust the subject as thoroughly as time and available facilities will permit.

At a purely legal level, the use of needles for insertion into the flesh for innumerable reasons has been sufficiently accepted and condoned both by the standards of the profession and by the courts throughout the United States as to make this type of procedure acceptable within the requirements of due care and proper administration. The long and satisfactory history of successful innoculations—vaccine, allergy shots, intravenous feeding, nerve blocks, pain killers, and many other uses—leaves no cause for concern when carefully performed, and the mere extension of this application of needles to other areas of the body and for other purposes creates no new problem beyond that which already exists.

Our courts have also held that a licensed and registered nurse who administered hypodermics under the immediate direction of an operating surgeon was not practicing medicine and could not be charged with violation of the law, nor could her supervising doctor be prosecuted for such supervision. Evidence showing that this was the uniform and accepted practice was admitted by the trial court as determinative on that point. One immediately wonders whether a registered nurse could administer acupuncture treatments to patients under the supervision of an attending doctor. This would depend upon the standards which had been adopted and put into practice in the community where the event occurred; at this stage of experimentation I would express the opinion that such practice could subject the parties to prosecution until acceptable guidelines were established and the nurse qualified herself thereunder.

What could constitute an act of negligence under these circumstances, and what dangers face the profession in embarking into this presently unexplored territory? The fact that there are reams of volumes covering the subject in a dozen countries does not meet the requirements of standard of care in this area, and therefore the forthcoming articles and papers on the subject, which will certainly follow this show of interest, will do much to establish the ground rules under which you can safely proceed. The provisions of law in force at the time of the commission of the act will also serve as a guideline as to the areas of involvement where one functions in conjunction with unlicensed persons.

California Ruling

On August 11, 1972, the Governor of California signed

Assembly Bill 1500 which adds Section 2145.1 to the Business and Professions Code, permitting the performance of acupuncture by an unlicensed person, alone or in conjunction with other forms of traditional Chinese medicine, when carried on in an approved medical school for the primary purpose of scientific investigation of acupuncture, providing that such procedures are carried on under the supervision of a licensed physician and surgeon.

A somewhat similar bill, A.B. 976, was presented to the legislature and passed by it, but vetoed by the governor. This bill would have permitted unlicensed persons to practice acupuncture under the direct supervision and diagnosis of a licensed dentist or physician or surgeon under certain conditions. This bill was not restricted to work carried on in an approved medical school. It is expected that this bill will be resubmitted in its original or in an amended form.

At the present time, it appears that technically most of the demonstrations and symposiums which are being conducted throughout the United States might well be in violation of existing provisions of the business and professions codes of the various states. However, this is primarily a matter for the concern of the law enforcement agencies; where the objectives are in the interests of scientific research, beneficial to the medical profession and the public at large, with no detrimental results to those participating, there appears to be no justification for harassment by the authorities. If, however, a complaint is received or pressure is applied by influential interests, one might expect the enforcement agencies to act in the manner.

From our reports to date, New York seems to be the most aggressive state in its prosecution of unlicensed acupuncturists. However, unless one is fully advised as to the facts surrounding each particular case and the motivation for prosecuting the individuals involved, it would be improper to comment or pass judgment at this time upon such activity.

The standard of care requirement will remain unchanged, and its application to the use of acupuncture will be the same as is presently applied to any other medical act. These standards will be set by your own members, and it will be they who have the responsibility of seeing to it that educational qualifications are established, seminars arranged, papers published, and other appropriate steps taken to afford doctors the opportunity of familiarizing themselves with all necessary phases of this subject. You will probably have to feel your way slowly but determinedly along this highway of endeavor until you have laid a sufficient foundation for your members to rely upon. In its initial stage of use as an anesthesia in uncomplicated cases, there appears to be little to concern oneself about along these lines, and it is primarily when one enters the more complex and far-reaching phases of acupuncture that greater skill and more knowledge will be required.

Viewing the cost of medical insurance, one wonders if anything can cause the skyrocketing rates to go any higher. Like automobile insurance and taxes, there seems to be no limit as to what devious minds can conjure up to increase the operation costs of your practice. Solely on the basis of extending your practice to include that of acupuncture, insurance men with whom I have discussed this subject see no justification for any increase based solely on your expansion of knowledge and the use of that knowledge in a new area. Costs of insurance, like many other economic facets of life, depend to a great degree on experience ratings, and I have found nothing from foreign countries to suggest that it will increase the rates here. So we come to grips with the last phase, namely, what specifically could go wrong to incur liability from this step.

Recognizing the accepted practice of insertion of needles for purposes of anesthesia, substituting the mere inserting of a needle for that of injecting a foreign substance into the body certainly does not increase the risk to a patient. Its use, if accepted, could afford the same immunity from pain, without the complications which have been known to follow a general anesthetic.

What if the patient suffers excruciating pain in the midst of an operation and emergency provisions have to be instituted? Proper precautionary measures would always require stand-by facilities which would be induced at once. Therefore, the only problem would be, What was the degree of extra pain the patient was forced to undergo, for how long a period, and to what extent, if any, did this event complicate, delay, or prevent his recovery or worsen his condition? The chances of this are extremely remote, particularly if the operating permit is carefully worded, the patient has a complete understanding of the possibilities facing him, and provided that he specifically requests this type of anesthesia. The legal aspects touching the issue of informed consent have been expanded by court decisions to warrant extra caution in advising patients of the probable consequences of any treatment so as to avoid a charge of battery or negligence.

Another potential, which always exists in any insertion of needles, is the possibility of hepatitis. However, proper sterilization would eliminate this chance of liability; despite the numerical increase in needle insertions, in the absence of negligence there is no danger from this source. A careful study of the acupuncture points and a knowledge of the human body will reveal to the prudent practitioner areas of danger where too deep penetration or improperly slanted or oriented needling may strike a vulnerable spot, and he will avoid these locations. An adequately prepared chart and designation of these areas will provide the necessary warning signals to the physician.

So the prospects are not nearly as serious as some have imagined. The unorthodox methods of diagnosis, from our point of view, including Chinese methods of pulse readings and sterilization, may differ considerably from the Western culture, and our methods will be judged solely by what standards are set up and followed or disobeyed by the doctor. The situation is as simple as that from the perspective of the law.

Another question is, What is the likelihood of American industry importing or manufacturing do-it-yourself kits and experimental dolls and making them available to the general public? And if it does so, what is the role of the medical profession in pointing out the dangers of self-infliction of needles and thus possibly neglecting required medical care in serious ailments?

In California and probably elsewhere throughout the United States these kits are being displayed and sold to members of the public who are experimenting upon their own bodies. While our attention has not been directed to any serious consequence as yet, the very nature of this practice could lead to disastrous results, and I believe that it is the duty of the medical profession to issue warnings to the public—through properly worded newspaper articles and reports in medical journals—of the possible dangers of any amateurish approach to this complicated phase of medical practice, which even the ordinarily qualified physician and surgeon in the United States is as yet unqualified to administer.

I believe that it is the duty of the medical fraternity not only to protect the public against charlatans and unqualified practitioners of the medical arts by which the public welfare might be adversely threatened, but also to make an unbiased and intelligently oriented thorough research into every phase of healing, regardless of the source from which it originates, in order to better educate the members of its own profession as to newly discovered ancient or current methods whereby doctors can better serve their patients and discharge their responsibility to those whose lives and welfare are placed in their hands in utmost confidence.

In conclusion I would like to speak about the usual transition of the position of the physician as regards acupuncture. He goes through a metamorphosis consisting of several stages, from bunking to belief.

Stage one is when first exposed to the word acupuncture—he smiles. Why does he smile? It's a comic technique—the needles, the chant, the spots, astrology . . . The next stage is when he is positive that acupuncture is a Chinese Communist political ploy. China has nothing to sell except acupuncture and ping-pong, and the Sinophiles are at it again. His third phase is that acupuncture is pure hypnosis. I hope we have dismissed that phase. His fourth is that maybe he ought to take a serious look at it. And the fifth and final phase will be its application in therapeutic practice.

Acupuncture, although it's supposed to help *eliminate* pain, has had a very painful introduction into American medicine, but will probably follow the French pattern. In France, in 1930, the arrival of the ancient Chinese healing art was greeted with skepticism and opposition. At that time there wasn't even the subject of hypnosis to which they could relate it, since that too was in disrepute. However, today acupuncture is an accepted part of the French medical curriculum and is taught and practiced throughout the country. Other European countries have followed this pattern as well.

Dr. Ilza Veith, writing in the *JAMA*, says the reason for this is that over the millenia of medical history innumerable theoretical therapeutic systems have been based on different theories as to the causation of disease. When the true nature of the illness has become established, the systems have in great part fallen by the wayside. True, an occasional one has persisted because of merits it possessed that were incidental to the theory upon which it was based. The medical historian wondering as to the fate of acupuncture in this context sees that it has survived.

CHAPTER XIV

A MODEL FOR MAKING ACUPUNCTURE CONSISTENT WITH WESTERN CONCEPTS OF BIOLOGICAL INFORMATION PROCESSING

Pal Greguss, Ph.D.

Research Professor at the Department of Ophthalmology, New York Medical College, New York, New York

Presented at the NIH Acupuncture Research Conference, Bethesda, Maryland, February 28-March 1, 1973.

Introduction

In dealing with the pressing problems of acupuncture that confront our contemporary Western traditional scientific strategies, the key to effective action is the development of a clear and realistic picture of what is really going on. Our present knowledge on this subject is, however, a large number of fragmentary pictures that can rarely be pieced together to form any coherent overall picture. The approach and language used in describing events is so different in the Western and Oriental biomedical usage that scientists from both sides do not realize that in reality they are talking about the same problem.

Since the time available is very restricted, I wish to show this only in one or two cases. For example, in most Western literature dealing with acupuncture, *Yang* and *Yin* is translated as "positive" and "negative." This associates in our minds something opposing, such as positive and negative electricity, positrons and electrons, etc. Further, we are unintentionally considering these principles as notions which can and/or may exist separately too. The original concept of *Yang* and *Yin* is, however, quite different. *Yang* and *Yin* are namely in the same relationship as a young girl and an old lady. An optical picture of both is simultaneously projected onto our retina, but we cannot recognize them simultaneously, and neither the girl nor the lady can be seen if the "other" is not there. Why?

Before answering the question, let us first consider the perhaps most misunderstood and misinterpreted meaning of *qi* (*chi*), which is generally described as live energy—*vis vitalis*—which flows from organ to organ through the network of elements beneath the skin called *chinglo*, or meridians. Since *qi*, as an energy form, cannot be identified with any known energy form, most Western physicians still view with disdain the claims made for acupuncture as a pain reliever or as a curing method, and nobody can really blame them.

The picture changes dramatically, however, if *qi* is not translated as "life energy" but is identified with "information," which flows from organ to organ through information channels called—if you wish—*chinglo* or meridians. This switch is not at all, though it may appear at first, a play on words, but is a very important fundamental recognition. The expression "information" is namely used in communication theory in a special way.[1] It is considered as determined by the probability of the state of some system and is invariably connected with a signal. It may be hard to believe, but it is also intimately connected to energy, i.e., to the energy capacity of the system.

Information transmission is always accomplished in a thermodynamic system having a temperature of T_0 and a minimum noise output of

$$Z = k.T_0 \, \Delta N$$

where $k = 1.38 \cdot 10^{-23}$ Ws/°K (k being the Boltzman constant and ΔN the bandwidth).

From this follows[2] that the energy to transmit one bit of information at room temperature is 3.10^{-21} Ws, i.e. transmission of information is an energy-consuming process. In other words, information is necessarily attached to a certain amount of energy, more correctly to an energy package. Therefore, transmission of information means energy flow. For preliminary examination of the model we wish to present, it is not of interest what type of energy it is, electrical, chemical, mechanical, etc. We have to keep in mind, however, that energy usually propagates in waveform. Further, according to Gabor's "expansion theorem,"[3] the information is carried not by rays, but by certain tubes of rays, whose cross section is determined by the wavelength of the information carrier.

There is no reason why we should not conceive the meridians of acupuncture as being Gabor-type information channels, although they are physiological entities which have, at least up till now, proved elusive to the anatomist. But this type of situation is well known from zoology, embryology, and paleontology. No anatomical evidence can be found—with the instrumentation available at present—for a given physiological function in one species, but the same function can be traced in other species anatomically too. So, e.g., the acousto-biliary reflex seems to be physiological in man, but can be traced anatomically only in a fish called Alosa Finata.[4]

We believe that an approach to the problems of acupuncture from this point of view will lead to answers which are more acceptable for Western-minded scientists. The scope of this presentation is, therefore, to start from these recognitions and to build up a model that defines pain in a way that both the Western practice of pain relief and the acupuncture treatment of pain can be interpreted.

The Bioholographic Model

Before discussing this model, two very important remarks have to be made. First, this model contains only those function groups which are necessary to describe pain-generating and pain-relieving processes, and it does not claim morphological equivalent, though it can lend insight to neurophysiological or experimental psychological events. Further, it is a deep model in the sense defined by Bross,[5] that is, it describes events at a level that is *not* directly observable. But it can be developed to a "deep mathematical model" in which the chain of events described in the model comprises both deep events and surface events, i.e., event chains which comprise only observable events.

Since, as we have seen, information is attached through signals to an energy package, which is, however, propagating in a wave form, the recording, storage and/or processing of the information pattern necessitates *simultaneous* recording of the *amplitude* and *phase* of the wavefront. And at this point, it seems that we are running into trouble, since all known biological energy receptors—but anorganic ones too—are sensitive only to the amplitude and not to phase relations. Yet everyday evidence shows that biological systems do process phase information since, for example, they move in 3-D space.

At the present stage of our knowledge, a simultaneous processing of phase and amplitude bound information can only be achieved by using principles related to holography, first described by Gabor just 25 years ago.[6]

At this spot, however, we have to emphasize that when setting up our model we are understanding under holography a principle, a new law of nature, similar to that of general relativity, and not a technical tool which allows us to record and reconstruct 3-D pictures.

The ingenious recognition of Gabor was that phase information can be processed as amplitude information—i.e., processed by square law detectors—simultaneously with other amplitude information if a well-defined coherent "reference background" is added to it, which then transforms the phase relations into proportional amplitude relations in a reversible way. Gabor called the result of this operation a "hologram," expressing the fact that it contains all information.

The principles of holographic information processing can easily be understood from a vector diagram. To the amplitude information and phase information φ, a coherent reference background A is added, and the resulting $A^2 \sim a^2 \sim 2Aa\cos\varphi$ amplitude contains, in a reversible form, both the amplitude and phase information. If this information is needed, it can be recovered in the original form by subtracting the reference background from the recorded amplitude value.

This is the process on which our model of biological information processing is based. Because the model has been described in detail in the Proceedings of the Seminar in Depth on Holography, 1971, I shall describe it only as far as it is necessary to understand how it can be applied to acupuncture.

The model starts from the recognition that the information (sensory) flow originating from both the outside world and from the living system itself is processed in information patterns, which are gated by a function group A. This information (stimulus) pattern can be described by the function f(x,y), where x,y are the characteristic coordinates of the information pattern. To process this pattern, which contains amplitude and phase information, a coherent reference background is needed (R). The question arises: From where can we expect such a coherent reference background?

Our answer is: from a part of the all neural activity of the living system.

It is known that events within the nerve cells maintain a quasi-constant level of sensitivity of the nerve substrate. This is shown by the constant activity of the brain. These activities can be kept apart from sensing activities in the same receptor caused by external stimuli, though, at the same time they are influenced by external and internal stimuli.[7]

It is, indeed, very difficult to recognize in this consideration the coherent reference background needed for a holographic model as long as we do not realize that the reference background has not to be devoid of information necessarily, if this information may be disregarded during the reconstruction of the information pattern. This, however, means that it is often difficult to distinguish between information stimulus and reference background. Indeed, these two may change their respective roles depending upon which information is actually needed.

Let us now recall what we said about the relation of *Yang* and *Yin*. It is not at all difficult to recognize that in both cases the same principles are involved: though both—*Yang* and *Yin*, girl and lady, respectively—are present, only one "acts" (can be seen), the other loses its "identity," but the roles can be switched. In other words, according to our model, *Yang* represents the reference background to process *Yin* information patterns, and *Yin* represents the reference background for *Yang* information patterns. But how does this relate to pain and its treatment?

Pain = Lack of Coherence

According to our model, a system is living and stays alive as long as it can handle—process—*all* the information patterns it receives, independently of their origin. Processing information patterns means, however, for the organism to be able to provide a given amount of coherence from its all-neural activity. If, however, the degree of coherence needed to process a given information pattern is not met—i.e., the signal-to-noise ratio is not adequate—the organism experiences pain. In other words, pain is a need for coherence, and it falls in the same category as hunger or sexual drive.

It follows from our model that there are two ways to eliminate pain. One is to cut off the information channel so that *no information processing* is needed. And this is the idea behind all kinds of pain treatment generally accepted today. How deeply this concept is innervated in our thinking can be seen from the fact that even when we try to explain acupuncture anesthesia, we develop a "gate control" concept, and when this does not explain how acupuncture needles stuck in the face would reduce pain in surgery of the abdomen, or how needles inserted in the arms would permit painless dental extraction, we "improve" our concept by putting a second gate in the model and wondering why it does not work.

According to our model, pain sensation can be eliminated by providing the necessary coherence needed to process the information pattern in question. And this is what happens during acupuncture anesthesia. The inserted needles and their vibrations are information signals which, when properly applied, improve coherence *in the region* where it is required by the information pattern to be processed. Therefore, contrary to general anesthesia, acupuncture in no way diminishes other aspects of the patient's consciousness.

Summary

In such a short time I could naturally give only a very brief description of our model of biomedical information processing, and how it can be applied to acupuncture. I wish, however, to point out that we are steadily refining our model, and my collaborators in Budapest have started a computer simulation of this bioholographic model of acupuncture; we hope to have results in the near future, which will allow us to determine where to insert the needles if we wish to restore coherence to relieve pain. This we hope will not only lead to a better understanding of acupuncture, but will also help "to separate acupuncture from quackpuncture," to quote Professor Kao.

REFERENCES

1. Greguss, P.: Bioholography. Proceedings Developments in Holography, SPIE 25, 55-87, 1971.
2. Marko, H., Neuburger, E.: Uber gerichteten Grossen in der Informationstheorie. Arch. Electr. Ubertragung 21:61-69, 1967.
3. Gabor, D.: Associative holographic memories. IMB J. Research & Development 13:156-159, 1969.
4. Mann, F.: The morphology of the gall bladder meridian. Lecture given at the Societe d'acupuncture, Paris, November, 1960.

5. Bross, J.D.J.: Scientific strategies in human affairs: use of deep mathematical models. Trans. New York Acad. Sci. 34:187-199, 1972.
6. Gabor, D.: A new microscopic principle. Nature 161:777-778, 1948.
7. Smolyaninov, V.A.: Some properties of the organization of cerebellar cortex. Ed. J.M. Gelfand, Nauka, Moscow, 1966.

CHAPTER XV

THE NIH ACUPUNCTURE RESEARCH STUDY

Howard P. Jenerick, Ph.D.
National Institute of General Medical Sciences

Background

Following a series of meetings sponsored by the Fogarty International Center of the National Institutes of Health, which covered the general subject of medicine and public health in the People's Republic of China, the traditional practice of acupuncture was singled out for further attention. In July, 1972, a special *ad hoc* advisory committee was appointed and met to consider the many suggested uses of acupuncture. This committee, whose membership included internationally recognized experts in the fields of anesthesiology, neurology, physiology, and psychology, recommended that the most valuable first approach to acupuncture in the United States would be studies on its use for surgical anesthesia and for the alleviation of chronic pain syndromes. Of particular interest were its mode of action and its relative effectiveness as compared to well-established forms of medical therapy.

Research Conference

At the request of the committee, all U.S. medical schools were also surveyed to determine if there was a significant research effort already underway. A total of 26 medical schools and universities responded affirmatively, and a conference was convened among those individuals so involved. At this conference, which was held on February 28 and March 1, 1973, 45 separate reports were presented.

Most of the reported research on acupuncture was in chronic pain treatment. Several reports were also included on the use of transcutaneous peripheral nerve or dorsal column stimulators for chronic pain. A number of minor surgical procedures, including dental applications, were also conducted under acupuncture anesthesia. Other applications included treatment of drug withdrawal symptoms, treatment of sensorineural deafness, and treatment of postoperative pain and ileus. Data were also presented from physiological and neurophysiological studies of the acupuncture effect in animals or on human volunteers. These studies also included attempts to identify the location and measure the properties of skin acupuncture points with various electrical instruments.

Summary of Conference

Based on the results presented at the conference, the NIH *ad hoc* Committee on Acupuncture concluded that acupuncture does produce effects which are of interest, and that it holds some promise as an anesthetic for some surgical operations and for the treatment of some acute and chronic painful conditions. It was not possible to even speculate on how acupuncture works or to say how well it compares with drug-induced anesthesia or with well-established procedures for treating pain. It was agreed that acupuncture is no panacea, and that many more well-designed and well-controlled studies are needed before it could be considered for wide use in clinical practice in the United States.

RESEARCH SUMMARIES

Chronic Pain: Acupuncture

Clinical investigators at eight separate pain clinics reported on acupuncture versus placebo treatments of acute and chronic pain in over 400 patients. Individual complaints and diagnoses ranged over a wide spectrum including phantom limb pain, causalgia and other neuropathy, headache and migraine, rheumatoid and osteo-arthritis pain, musculo-skeletal pain, etc. In many of these instances, the patients had experienced failure with conventional treatments, and had been referred to the pain clinic by their original attending physicians. While many of these studies had not evolved to the point where strictly controlled or double blind procedures were employed, several investigators presented data indicating that acupuncture at traditional or recommended points was at least twice as effective in relieving pain than was acupuncture needling at nearby control points. Standard syringe needles (27-30 gauge) were reputedly similar in effectiveness to acupuncture needles. The latter, however, do not have cutting edges.

On the order of 60% of all patients reported "good" to "excellent" relief from their pain for periods ranging from hours to months. Results varied according to the underlying pathology. The best outcome was obtained with self-limiting diseases, although some conditions of long standing (*i.e.*, chronic headache, arthritis, low back pain) also responded well. As a rough rule, joint pain responded better in lightly loaded joints such as shoulder or neck than it did if located in the hip or knee. There was enough variation in the practices of the individual clinics, coupled with relatively small numbers of patients within each diagnostic category, to preclude any firm conclusion about the effectiveness of acupuncture for any particular application.

Most of the investigators agreed that the results obtained after the first treatment of any one patient would not predict the eventual outcome of a series of further treatments. Some patients responded eventually; others never did, for no obvious reasons.

By and large, the data presented consisted of individual patients' verbal reports that they felt better or were able to decrease or stop their regular medication. One clinic dealing with rheumatoid arthritis, neck and back pain, and headache also monitored blood pressure, skin temperature, and peripheral blood flow during the treatment period. While systolic pressures might drop 10-30 mm H_g with acupuncture, diastolic pressure and pulse rate changes were minimal. However, vasodilation in the treated extremities often occurred, and if peripheral circulation had been poor, there was a resulting reduction of edema and raised skin temperatures. Concomitantly, pain was reduced, and the patient obtained more joint motion. In two patients with an established diagnosis of reflex sympathetic dystrophy of the upper extremities, as circulation was improved, remineralization of carpal bones was demonstrated by X-ray. The investigator stated his belief that some of the long-range clinical improvements were secondary to these acupuncture-induced changes in circulation. This study also included a comparison between the effectiveness of acupuncture treatment in individuals and their scores in a test of hypnotizability. No direct correlation was found.

One study which attracted much interest was designed as a pure placebo test. Twelve out of 18 patients with chronic pain, predominantly in the low back, reported relief when treated by a physician, admittedly naive in acupuncture, who placed needles at random subcutaneously and spent about ½ hour in sympathetic discussion with each patient.

The discussions following each report tended to deal with possible alternate explanations for the observed results, ranging from placebo or novelty effect to suggestibility or hypnosis. In the absence of tightly controlled studies, admittedly difficult to devise, no consensus on a true, therapeutic effect for acupuncture could be reached. It also appeared on the basis of verbal reports that acupuncture therapy is rapidly evolving in the People's Republic of China and that many of their classical procedures are being discarded. Hence, it is often difficult to obtain reliable information on accepted, effective treatment procedures.

Chronic Pain—Electrical Stimulation

Reports from four neurosurgical investigations, using cutaneous or implanted electrodes, were presented on a total of 600 patients with intractable or chronic pain. Diagnoses were similar to the acupuncture series. Results were also similar, ranging from 60-70% of the patients reporting good to excellent pain relief during application of weak electrical stimuli to the skin over peripheral nerves, to implanted cuff electrodes on peripheral nerve trunks, or to electrodes implanted in the dorsal columns. Some of the patients remained pain-free for hours after the stimulation period. Medication use decreased, and activity levels improved. Failures were traced to electrode mechanical problems or invasion of connective tissue. One investigator reported his belief that there may be an element of suggestibility in these results, since the degree of effectiveness in a series of patients dropped off from 60% to 40% when a skeptical operator was put in charge.

Experimental Pain and Acupuncture

Another series of studies concerned the possible effects of acupuncture on pain experimentally induced in animals and human volunteers. Accepting the difficulties of identifying in lightly anesthetized animals specific nerve tracts subserving pain, or associating neuronal activity within the central nervous system with a pain "sensation," various investigators reported modifications in unit activity in thalamus or cord, cortical evoked potentials, and vocalization during acupuncture stimulation. In several cases, normal activity or pre-test behavior returned 30-50 minutes after acupuncture stimulation ceased. In an extensive series on rabbits, tested by a vigorous skin pinch, various needling sites were evaluated for their ability to produce skin anesthesia. Electo-acupuncture was employed rather than manual twirling. The area involved and the time of onset varied according to needle location and stimulation frequency.

Normal volunteers were exposed to ischemic limb pain, pin prick, or electric stimulation of dental pulp. Acupuncture delayed the onset of various levels of ischemic pain similar to a 10-mmg dose of morphine, while a placebo dose or needling at a non-acupuncture point did not. In another study, only one subject out of five developed an analgesia to dental pulp stimulation after acupuncture needling in the ipsilateral hand (at the dorsal, first interosseus web or *hoku* point). Comments were made by others that additional needles might be required, as if the analgesia was dose- or needle-related. On the other hand, a similar study employing the *hoku* point obtained analgesia to pin prick in the oral cavity and in the treated arm in 4 of 6 subjects. As needling proceeded, the analgesic area gradually extended further and further up the arm, although the maximum area involved varied among subjects. In yet another study, mild electrical stimuli at 45 or 250 cps. were applied to a needle electrode placed near the ulnar nerve. Definite analgesia, without loss of proprioception, developed along the ulnar distribution with some spreadout to the hand and outlasted the stimulation period by about 8 minutes. In contrast, if the stimuli were applied to a subcutaneously implanted needle electrode in the forearm, no analgesia was demonstrable.

Acupuncture Analgesia in Surgery

The predominantly reported use of acupuncture analgesia was in dental surgery of various types ranging from deep scaling and cystectomy to extraction of impacted teeth (one of which required mallet and chisel). Of 37 total cases discussed, 8 experienced pain breakthrough and procedures were continued under local anesthesia. Several patients reported no postoperative pain for up to 12 hours and did not use analgesics. Most were pleased with the outcome and were willing to undergo acupuncture in the future.

A variety of other surgical procedures was also attempted under acupuncture analgesia, such as tonsillectomy, herniorrhaphy, Colle's fracture reduction, and repair of a recurring shoulder dislocation. Of 7 such cases, one fracture reduction was unsuccessful, and 2 herniorrhaphy patients experienced discomfort and nausea when traction was applied to the spermatic cord. The latter cases also reported postoperative pain relief for 4-6 hours.

No other problems or complications were reported. However, the induction period may range up to 30 minutes, and if manual stimulation is employed, several physician-anesthesiologists may be needed. (A useful alternative is electro-acupuncture, since a number of sites can be handled by one operator.) Apprehensive patients usually do not respond, and pre-selection and initial interviews are usually required.

One interesting subject that was not extensively pursued was the use of acupuncture to induce labor as well as to control obstetric pain in four deliveries. This raised the possibility of using acupuncture at special points for therapeutic abortion.

Discussion again revolved around the alternate possibility of hypnosis as the underlying "analgesic," without any definite conclusion. It did seem as if there might be a hypnotic overlay to acupuncture analgesia, since subjects who rate very low on hypnotizability are poor candidates for acupuncture analgesia. Those who rate very high, may or may not be. Predictability of success on the whole is perhaps 80%, which poses obvious problems to the patient, the anesthesiologist, and the surgeon. None of the anesthesiologists using acupuncture felt it would be widely accepted as a surgical analgesic in the U.S.

Other Reported Studies

A few cautious, preliminary attempts have been made in this country to assess the utility of some of the traditionally recommended applications. In a series of 40 post-laparotomy patients, acupuncture was employed to relieve distension; simultaneously, the incidence of ileus dropped to a very low figure. This observation was confirmed by animal work, wherein acupuncture in vagotomized rabbits increased GI motility and promoted defecation. This report prompted a neurosurgeon to remark that in 100 patients treated for postoperative pain with continuous electrical stimulation by cutaneous electrodes placed along the incision under the surgical dressing, postoperative ileus dropped to only 2%. In a matched series of untreated patients, similarly operated on for gastrectomy, cholecystectomy, or thoractomy, the incidence was 25%.

Another application consisted of electrostimulation by skin electrodes of acupuncture points around the pinna for sensorineural deafness. The schedule consisted of five daily treatments a week for six weeks. About one-half of a randomly selected group of 70 patients so treated gradually developed a moderate improvement in word recognition tests. There was no change in pure tone thresholds and no patient noted subjective improvements after one treatment. The hypothesis was advanced that stimulation improved circulation in the inner ear which assisted hair cell metabolism. If treatments ceased, the improvements were said to be gradually lost over 20-30 days.

Finally, one case was mentioned in which acupuncture was helpful in controlling withdrawal symptoms in a drug addict. The suggestion was then advanced, as supported by other data on an acupuncture effect on heart rate, blood pressure and circulation, GI function, etc., that acupuncture works by activating portions of the autonomic nervous system to ameliorate such withdrawal symptoms as sweating, tearing, vomiting, cramps, tachycardia, etc.

Physiology of Acupuncture

There was a relative paucity of data available on physiologic correlates of acupuncture as compared to the expressed need for such information. Reference has already been made above to shifts in peripheral blood flow, skin temperature, GI function, heart rate, etc. Remarks made during discussion also indicated that acupuncture-induced shifts can occur in EEG, plethysmographic pulse wave, etc. The points used were said to consistently affect a particular function, yet if needling was applied to a control or non-acupuncture point located 1 cm. distant, no effect was observed.

This in turn led to a discussion of the location, identification, and reality of acupuncture points. During the conference, at least seven research groups reported experiments using various electrical devices, which measure skin resistance or potential, to locate positions where skin properties were altered. These loci were more or less punctate and similarly located on the right versus the left side of any individual and from day to day in the same individual. Locations often agreed among individuals (including children and adults) and with published traditional acupuncture charts. They bore no relation to major blood vessels in the extremities. A 1972 report from the People's Republic of China was then read into the record and stated that about one-half the known acupuncture points are located right over various nerves and the rest lie within half a centimeter of one or another nerve. Anatomical and histological studies could not confirm the presence of meridian channels or vessels, and the Chinese have concluded that acupuncture acts in fact on the nervous system. Anesthesiologists at the conference confirmed this generally, in the sense that they recognized many acupuncture loci as sites where nerve blocks are performed in Western medical practice.

One preliminary report concerned the possible alteration of the properties of acupuncture points with disease, as has been traditionally claimed. Although the investigators themselves expressed caution in reaching any conclusion, in six patients following a cholecystectomy, several points on the traditional gallbladder meridian on the right side were more easily located (that is, their electrical properties were more markedly altered) than symmetrical points on the left side or in six other patients following a herniorrhaphy.

General Information

A number of related issues have come to the attention of the study committee. These were received as information only and their inclusion here is in that context and does not represent any endorsement or confirmation.

The Office of Medical Devices of the Food and Drug Administration, exercising its responsibilities under the labeling act, has stated that acupuncture devices must be labeled to indicate that they are experimental devices limited to investigational use by or under the direct supervision of a licensed medical or dental practitioner. Further details are published in the *Federal Register,* vol. 38, No. 46 (page 6419), Friday, March 9, 1973.

In virtually every state that has taken a formal position, there is no doubt that acupuncture is viewed as a medical procedure which can be practiced legally only by or under the supervision of licensed practitioners. One state (California) permits acupuncture by non-M.D.'s if engaged in approved research projects conducted within medical schools. Since each state exercises its own responsibility to regulate medical practice, there is no federal role, and further clarification must be sought locally.

Status Report on Acupuncture Research

Report of a Workshop sponsored by the National Institute of General Medical Sciences, March 14, 1975.

A workshop was sponsored by the National Institute of General Medical Sciences to review the current status of acupuncture research projects conducted under NIH grant support or by NIH intramural scientists. Current studies are in various stages of completion, and no final reports are available. Scientists expert in anesthesiology, clinical medicine, and neurophysiology were also present. A summary of the conference follows:

In several studies, acupuncture seemed to be about as effective as doses of mild analgesics such as codeine, nitrous oxide gas, and morphine in reducing or controlling various types of experimental pain such as that caused by electric shock, heat lamp, or ice cold water. However, in one study there was no observable effect of acupuncture on painful electric shock.

In a study of postoperative pain, when used on 20 patients following multiple tooth extractions, the pain-relieving effect of acupuncture came on more rapidly than that of codeine, a widely used oral analgesic, although its effective duration was shorter. The investigators noted that a mix of the two procedures provided a better clinical result, that is, a more rapid onset of pain relief from the acupuncture and a more prolonged period of relief from the codeine.

Several studies also demonstrated an appreciable psychological element in the pain-relieving effects of acupuncture, in addition to its apparent direct effect on the neurosensory system. This did not seem to be an unusual result, since other procedures—for example, nitrous oxide gas—caused similar changes in a patient's expectations or belief, which tended to reduce or even abolish painful sensations. In fact, several groups reported that hypnosis was more effective than acupuncture in controlling experimental pain.

In another investigation, only one of 15 tested patients with diagnosed essential hypertension showed a mild decrease (10 mm Hg) of blood pressure after prolonged acupuncture treatments.

In a general discussion of these reports, the panel emphasized that any conclusions about the effectiveness of acupuncture based on the work in progress would be premature. The evidence presented indicated that the response to acupuncture, like that to many other treatment procedures, may be dependent on a patient's attitudes and expectations, which, in turn, are important in the perception of pain. The preliminary results, suggesting that acupuncture can act as a mild analgesic, serve more to underscore the puzzle of pain rather than demonstrate the effectiveness of any procedure intended for its treatment. Although continued work on acupuncture is to be encouraged as a non-drug approach to pain control, the panel stressed the need for studies directed at the phenomenon of pain itself.

These statements and opinions do not necessarily represent the official position of the NIH. Responsibility for any errors in summarizing data and statements from individual investigators or research teams likewise lies with the author.

APPENDIX i

ELECTRICAL ACUPUNCTURE

GLOSSARY OF ELECTRICAL TERMS

Your reading in acupuncture analgesia will be helped by understanding the following terms:

Ammeter. A device for measuring the flow of electrical current.
Ampacity. The current-carrying capacity in amperes.
Ampere. The unit of measurement of current. *See Ohm's Law.*
Anode. Positively charged electrode.
Capacitance. The ability to retain an electrical charge.
Cathode. Negatively charged (ground) electrode.
Conductance. The ability of a material to conduct electricity, measured in mhos; the opposite of resistance.
Electron. Negative charge of electricity.
Hertz (Hz). A unit of measurement of frequency; one hertz equals one cycle per second; named after the German physicist Heinrich Hertz who made the first successful radio transmission.
Impedance. Interference with the passage of some form of physical energy through a medium. Electrical impedance refers to the interference with the passage of electrical current through a conducting medium. If a signal is a truly direct current signal, impedance would be synonymous with resistance. Since many physiologic signals, although of direct current nature, occur repetitively with fairly rapid frequency, the impedance of the tissues through which they pass would be a factor of the resistance, capacitance, physiologic effects such as electrical anesthesia; capacitance and conductance would assume major factors in the impedance of the tissues through which such a current is made to pass.

Isolation Transformer. A transformer which inductively couples its secondary winding to the grounded feeder system that energizes its primary winding, thereby isolating the secondary winding from ground potential.

Macroshock. Electrical shock produced by current in the *millampere* range penetrating the intact skin.

Mho. A unit of measurement of electrical conductance; the reciprocal of ohm.

Microshock. Electrical shock produced by current in the *microampere* range, introduced into the body of the electrically susceptible patient by the conductive pathway to the patient's heart.

Ohm. A unit of measurement of electrical resistance.

Ohm's Law. The law expressing the relationship between resistance, voltage, and current flowing through a circuit; one ohm of resistance will cause a voltage drop of one volt when one ampere of current is flowing through the resistance. Stated by George S. Ohm, German physicist, in 1827.

Power. The capacity for performing work; energy generated or consumed per unit time. *See Watt.*

Resistance. In physics, refers to any modality which opposes motion; electrical resistance is a property of a conductor which opposes motion; electrical (i.e., electrical current) through it; resistance is measured in ohms.

Risk Class 1 Patient. Patients who have no intentional contact with electrodes, ambulatory patients, and many bed patients with minimal contact with electrical appliances.

Risk Class 2 Patient. Patients, ambulatory and nonambulatory, subject to diagnostic or therapeutic procedures involving electrical appliances.

Risk Class 3 Patient. Patients with externalized conductors, diagnostic catheters, or other direct electrical contact with the conduction system of the heart.

Semiconductor. A material that will pass more current than an insulator but not as much as a conductor. Germanium and silicon are the two materials now being utilized for the manufacture of semiconductors. By imposing the proper electrical charge on a certain phase of the semiconductor, the conductance through the semiconductor is altered.

Solid State Device. A component of electronic equipment consisting of a solid block of special material designed to handle electrical signals in a special way. The transistor is an example of a solid state device. *See Semiconductor.*

Transistor. A semiconductor which possesses the same functions as the vacuum tube.

Volt. A unit of measurement of difference in electrical potential; named after the Italian physicist Volta.

Voltage. A difference in electrical potential in volts; electromotive force.

Voltmeter. A device designed to measure voltage.

Watt. A unit of power; part of the metric system of measurement. It represents one *joule* of energy being converted or consumed *per second.* Electrical appliances are rated in watts. One watt of electrical power is the amount dissipated through a resistance of one ohm when the current flow is one ampere.

Above definitions taken from Dornette, ed. *Monitoring in Anesthesia,* Philadelphia: F. A. Davis Company, 1973.

Electrical acupuncture is not an ancient Chinese art. As we have stated repeatedly, it began in China around 1958, with the attachment of electricity from a small stimulator to the acupuncture needles already in place.

Surprisingly enough, there was a group of electrical acupuncturists in Japan as early as 1950, under the aegis of Dr. Yoshiro Nakatani, who claim to have preceded the Chinese. Nonetheless, whichever national group was first, an electrical instrument will undoubtedly form the basis for modern American acupuncture. Let us start with a description and understanding of these machines before proceeding further. The Chinese 626, one of the first in this country, is essentially a portable battery-powered electrical stimulator applied to the skin through flexible conductors and miniature electrical clips. The wires are clipped directly onto acupuncture needles or deep pins as electrodes. (See Schematic.)

The instrument delivers at its output a negative going pulse utilizing pulse time modulation (abbr. PTM).

The main controls over the output are: (1) a five-position pulse modulation selector, and (2) a variable potentiometer for pulse amplitude or intensity. The instrument also contains a moving coil meter with an arbitrary scale. The meter is used to indicate electrode conduction and to monitor pulse intensity, as well as to act as a battery check. A second 9-volt battery automatically takes over the function of the circuit when the first battery delivers less than 5 volts.

The essential output pulse train, which is relative to all five positions of the selector, are pulses of constant shape and duration. Analysis of a single pulse shows an exponential wave shape with a rise time of 5 microseconds, and decay or fall time of 100 microseconds. Essential width of pulse is 70 microseconds. The pulse contains 10% quantization distortion of instantaneous wave. The resultant unmodulated repetition rate of pulse train is 50 pulses per second.

The peak-to-peak voltage of output pulses varies from 10 volts minimum to 160 volts maximum. This holds true for all five positions of the modulation selector. In vitro these peak-to-peak voltage measurements were made with minimum loading. Under actual clinical usage of the instrument, of course, the measurable peak-to-peak voltage at clips will be reduced somewhat by skin impedance.

A special electrode provides a frequency of from 3,000-6,000 Hertz.

Examination of pulse modulation and effect:

With selector in position 1, time modulation is employed. An oscilloscope display shows pulse interruption. An oscilloscope with calibrated sweep time presents a pulse train of 2-second duration, followed by a 1-second interval at zero amplitude. Each pulse train has a rapid exponential rise to desired amplitude, and a rapid exponential fall. Thus, the envelope pulse is 20 pulses per minute. The exponent of each envelope pulse is 50 pulses per second. This is variable from 10 to 160 volts peak-to-peak volts. This position and output results in the stimulation of human tissue to the point of analgesia or hypesthesia.

Examination of modulation selector position 2:

An oscilloscope display shows a different time modulation. A pulse train of 50 pulses per second for duration of ½ second, alternating with a pulse omission time of 1.5 seconds, the envelope pulse produced being 40 pulses per minute, each pulse envelope containing approximately 25 separate pulses, with amplitude variable from 10 to 160 volts peak-to-peak. This position and output, when applied to the skin by electrodes, particularly to the cranial area, has been capable of producing a drowsiness or somnolence similar to that state produced by mild to moderate hypnosis. This is useful in cases of mild insomnia, acute anxiety, and a variety of minor psychiatric disorders.

Examination of modulation selector positions 3, 4, and 5:

Again a very different time modulation in this position. A pulse rate of 50 pulses per second for a duration of 1.5 seconds, alternating with a pulse rate of 8 pulses per second, each pulse being of same wave shape and amplitude. This position and output, when applied to the skin or various parts of the human body, has been found to produce a tingling sensation of a stimulatory effect, which has been useful in restoring circulation and in helping deep muscle aches and pains.

Oscilloscope examination of modulation selector 4 shows a uniform pulse rate of 300 pulses per minute, each pulse being of uniform wave shape and having the same characteristics as previously described in the paragraph on single-pulse analysis. This position and output, when electrodes have been introduced into the skin, has been found to produce a state of stimulation and analgesia in tissue, localized to the area between the electrodes, useful in localized operative procedures of a superifical nature, such as the removal of warts, moles, and skin excrescences.

Oscilloscope display of position 5 shows a steady repetitive pulse at a frequency of 50 pulses per second with the same pulse characteristics as described above. This position and output has been found to be useful to conduct a train of impulses along the beta fibers and thus to produce a pain-blocking effect applicable in minor and major surgery of all types.

The electrodes on the machine are of several types. One resembles acupuncture needles that have been reduced in size by eliminating the handle customarily used for twisting and twirling. It resembles a modified pin such as is used in pinning. The second set of electrodes is disposable, spherical electrodes, used in conjunction with electrocardiographic fluid or jelly. The third set of electrodes resembles the foregoing electrodes except for the addition of a small pin-like attachment in the center in order to make contact with the alligator clamps more effective.

In 1972, in a transparent attempt to prevent acupuncture from being either practiced or researched, the Federal Drug Administration "embargoed" the importation of acupuncture needles from foreign sources. It was claimed that they were "improperly packaged and labeled."

This has resulted in the adaptation of other materials for use in acupuncture. Dr. Allen Russek at New York University's Institute for Rehabilitation used modified guitar strings and finds that they are quite effective. Other acupuncture researchers have gotten their supply of needles from the notions store (probably not the first time in the history of medical research!).

Testing with the ordinary superficial neurologic method of sharp and dull is frequently inadequate for an accurate appraisal of the degree of analgesia. Passing a pin through the skin is more appropriate, since the patient will feel but will not interpret this feeling as pain, since the pain pathway is overloaded.

Care must be taken that stainless steel needles are the materials which form the basis for the needle. The introduction of other metals in the manufacture of acupuncture needles may be the cause of serious damage, since under the impetus of an electrical charge the body will act as a galvanic cell, polarizing the acupuncture needles as they would electrodes, and depositing active metallic ions at the site of the puncture. This could easily result in a localized chemical burn, with necrotic tissue resulting from this burn difficult to heal and dangerous to the organism. One such burn was developed by an acupuncturist during his early days of experimentation, and he states that it took almost six months before his leg healed. Perhaps this anecdote illustrates why the Chinese insist that fledgling acupuncturists practice on themselves before venturing out into the foreign fields of medical practice.

In an effort to overcome this difficulty and improve on the Oriental techniques, a specially designed acupuncture needle has been produced in this country and will soon be marketed. It combines the best features of Chinese and American needleware. It is easy to sterilize, and provides the amateur acupuncturist with an important assist in that the handle makes it extremely simple to "screw" the needle into the skin without too much pain or difficulty.

Utilizing the machine and the needles makes effective electrical acupuncture a relatively painless and effective procedure. Standard acupuncture points may be employed, but if these yield no results then application of a little judgment will not hurt. The needles may be moved closer to the site of the affliction, and the latest model of the machine allows for the placement of two to six needles, reinforcing the basic technique by three. Two machines may be used, if one is not adequate, and any variation of acupuncture recipes may then be tried until a successful formula is devised.

Repeated applications are necessarily required in afflictions of long standing. One-treatment spontaneous "cures" have been demonstrated again and again, for which there is no scientific explanation other than on a strictly psychosomatic basis. Long-standing afflictions, such as one finds in the rheumatic and arthritic disease processes, have yielded to electric acupuncture after persistent efforts.

It is important that no guarantees or advance claims be provided by the practitioner, since the therapeutic effects are at best spotty and as yet uncontrolled. But there is no doubt that in many, many cases the machine works, and there is no greater gratification in medical practice than to have a patient unable to crawl up on the treatment bed before acupuncture and then airily walk out of your office with a spring in his step and a whole new outlook on life due to alleviation of the painful symptoms. This has happened many times, and the percentage seems to indicate that something other than hypnosis is at work.

The same apparatus is the one used in surgical and dental nerve-blocking. Here the traditional points are of exceptional value mainly because the points are out of range of the surgical field, and acupuncture therefore does not intrude on the surgeon's and surgical supervisor's sensibilities. For the lower abdomen, the traditional *pei ying, nienchu, tsusanli, hoku, yangpai,* and *yangtai* positions are all convenient puncture sites. Translated into our neurologic concept, this means that needles were placed in proximity to the supraorbital nerve, supratrochlear nerve, peroneal nerve, radial nerve (the apex of the web between the first and second metacarpals), infraorbital nerve, and greater auricular nerve. As is obvious, unless operation is taking place directly on these sites, all can be managed quite successfully without interfering with the procedure.

The characteristics of the electrical current needed to provide analgesia vary from patient to patient and from operation to operation. Several positions on the machine will work exceedingly well on one operation, only to fail in others; and here we must remember that the Chinese claim success in nine out of ten operations, the tenth one requiring conventional anesthesia. Perhaps it seems somewhat unscientific to rely on this hit-and-miss method of finding the ideal setting, but a small degree of advance preparation can eliminate this. The day before the operation, a test run with the patient and the machine should be arranged, thus accomplishing the double purpose of familiarizing the patient with the procedure and giving the anesthesiologist some advance warning of the degree of analgesia he can obtain. Experimentation with various settings can be effected at this time. The induction of analgesia will require a minimum of 15 to 30 minutes, not unlike the early days of ether induction. Appropriately enough, it can be managed in the same manner by desensitizing the patient in an induction room and not bringing him into the operating room until the analgesia is established. This system functions equally well in a dental office, and the dental surgeon need have no fear of over-anesthetizing his patient.

Federal Register, Vol. 38, No. 45 — Friday, March 9, 1973

ACUPUNCTURE DEVICES LABELING

Notice to Manufacturers, Packers and Distributors

The Commissioner of Food and Drugs is aware of the current interest in the United States surrounding the use of acupuncture needles, stimulators, and other accessories for medical purposes. Acupuncture paraphernalia are being imported into this country and are also being manufactured domestically for various medical uses, including the treatment and diagnosis of serious diseases, anesthesia and pain relief. These products are devices and must comply with all applicable provisions of the Federal Food, Drug and Cosmetic Act.

It is the position of the Food and Drug Administration that the safety and effectiveness of acupuncture devices have not yet been established by adequate scientific studies to support the many and varied uses for which such devices are being promoted, including uses for analgesia and anesthesia. Although various theories have been advanced as to how medical results can be obtained through the use of acupuncture, none has been proved or generally accepted, and there is a body of scientific opinion which questions the safety and effectiveness of acupuncture in many of the uses for which it is now being applied.

Under the Federal Food, Drug, and Cosmetic Act, all devices must be properly labeled to be in compliance with the law. Devices which are not safe for use by the laity, or for which adequate directions cannot be written for safe use by the laity, must be labeled as prescription devices and must be accompanied by labeling which provides the prescribing practitioner with adequate directions for their safe and effective use. Because the safety and effectiveness of acupuncture devices have not yet been adequately demonstrated, and labeling therefore cannot be devised, which would provide adequate directions for safe and effective use, they may not be labeled in accordance with the requirements for prescription devices as stated in 21 CFR 1.106(d). Until evidence is obtained demonstrating that acupuncture is a safe and effective medical technique, acupuncture devices must be limited to investigational or research use.

Current Food and Drug Administration regulations do not contain specific provisions governing the shipment of investigational devices in interstate commerce for clinical research or experimental use. The Commissioner of Food and Drugs is aware of the need for such regulations to provide adequate guidance as to the labeling for experimental devices to be used on human beings. Therefore, the Commissioner intends to publish at a later date proposed regulations which would govern all investigational devices. In the interim, this notice will apply to all acupuncture devices.

In order to establish guidelines under which manufacturers, packers, and distributors can properly label acupuncture devices for investigational use, the Food and Drug Administration met on September 22, 1972, with individuals concerned with the use of acupuncture in the United States. These included representatives of the States of California and New York, the city of New York, the American Society of Anesthesiologists, the National Institutes of Health, the Federation of State Medical Boards, the American Medical Association, medical practitioners, and the Food and Drug Administration Medical Device Advisory Committee. It was the consensus of this group that acupuncture devices should include this restriction in addition to other information.

Accordingly, the Commissioner of Food and Drugs concludes that until substantial scientific evidence is obtained by valid research studies supporting the safety and therapeutic usefulness of acupuncture devices, the Food and Drug Administration will regard as misbranded any acupuncture device shipped in interstate commerce if the following information does not appear in the labeling:

(a) The name of the device.

(b) The name and place of business of the manufacturer, packer, or distributor.

(c) An accurate statement of the quantity of the contents.

(d) The composition of the device and whether it is sterile, nonsterile, reusable, or disposable.

(e) The dimension or other pertinent physical characteristics of the device.

(f) The following statement: "Caution: Experimental device limited to investigational use by or under the direct supervision of a licensed medical or dental practitioner. This device is to be used only with informed consent under conditions designed to protect the patient as a research subject, where the scientific protocol for investigation has been reviewed and approved by an appropriate institutional review committee, and where conditions for such use are in accordance with State law."

Instructions for the use of the device for the purpose for which it is being investigated and, to the extent such information is known, any human hazards, contraindications, precautions, or side effects associated with its use, should be provided to researchers and investigators. The Food and Drug Administration, however, will regard as misbranded any acupuncture device shipped in interstate commerce if accompanied by claims of diagnostic or therapeutic effectiveness.

Pending promulgation of separate regulations for conducting clinical investigations of investigational devices, researchers and investigators shall assure adequate informed consent and institutional committee review for such investigations, utilizing as a guideline the standards established for investigational drugs in 21 CFR 130.37 and in Division 10, unit C of form FD-1571, in 21 CFR 130.3(a) (2).

Dated: February 21, 1973.

SHERWIN GARDNER,
Deputy Commissioner
of Food and Drugs.

(FR Doc. 73-4540 Filed 3-8-73; 8:45 am)

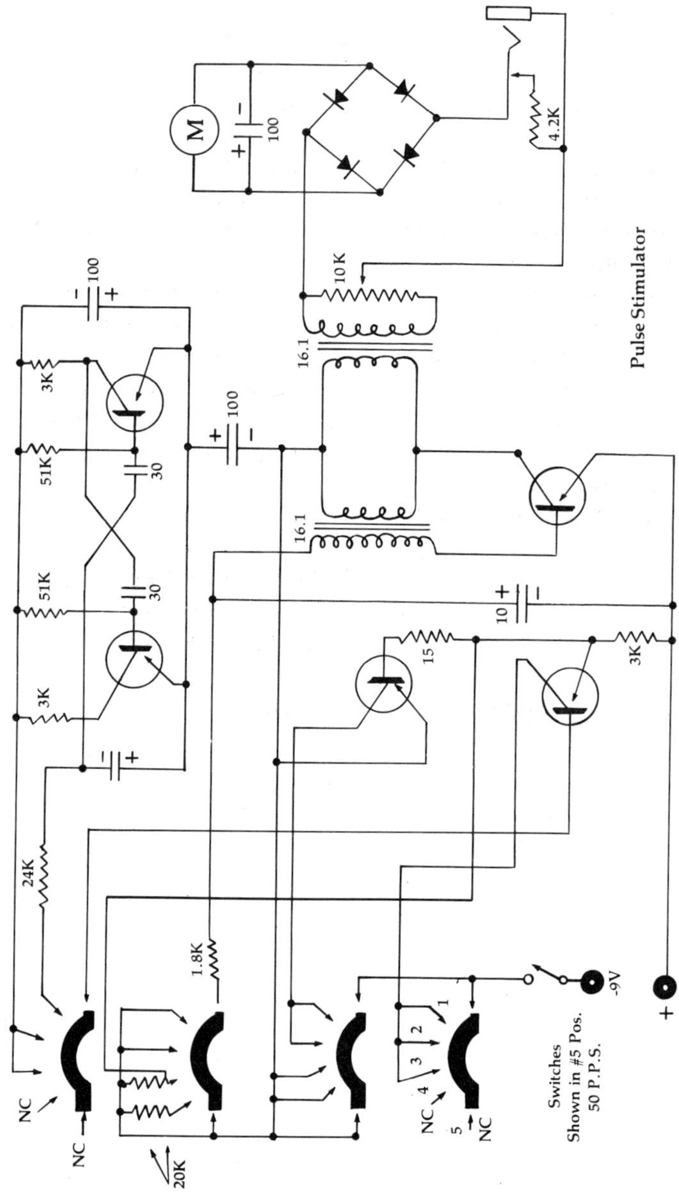

Schematic for a Pulse Generator Useful in Acupuncture

APPENDIX ii

RECOMMENDED FORMS AND PROCEDURES

REFUSAL TO SUBMIT TO TREATMENT

Date________________________________ Time A.M.____________
P.M.____________

I have been advised by Dr. ________________________________
that it is necessary for me to undergo the following treatment:

(*Describe operation or treatment*)

The effect and nature of this treatment have been explained to me.

Although my failure to follow the advice I have received may seriously imperil my life or health, I nevertheless refuse to submit to the recommended treatment. I assume the risks and consequences involved and release the above-named physician, the hospital and its staff from any liability.

Signed ________________________________

AUTHORIZATION FOR TREATMENT WITH PROCEDURE UNDER CLINICAL INVESTIGATION

Date_________________________________ Time A.M.___________
P.M.___________

I authorize Dr. ____________________________, the attending physician, to treat (*name of patient*) with the drug presently identified as ____________________________ for the following condition:

(*Describe symptoms of disease to be treated*)

It has been explained to me that the safety and usefulness of the procedure in the treatment of patients for the above condition are now being investigated and that the manufacturer (
) of the device is held blameless.

Signed______________________________

I, the undersigned, hereby give my voluntary consent for the administration of treatment by the method known as acupuncture. This technique is to be applied by or under the direction and supervision of Dr. __________________________, whom I hereby release from any responsibility.

Acupuncture has been explained to me as a medical treatment performed by the insertion of special needles (with or without the application of small pulses of electric current to the needles) through the skin into the underlying tissue at certain indicated points on the surface of the body, for the purpose of the alleviation or cure of painful bodily diseases and disorders for an undetermined time.

I have been made aware of the possibility of complications that may result from this procedure. These include: infection, ecchymoses, hemorrhages in the tissues, pain and discomfort, weakness, fainting, nausea, areas of anesthesia, needle breakage and its retention, and even aggravation of symptoms.

I am aware that the use of acupuncture to which I am consenting is not a common practice in this community. I accept the fact that there are no guarantees through the use of acupuncture.

Signed______________________________

Recommendations

Sometimes the refusal of a patient to submit to necessary surgery or treatment will result in serious injury or death. Under these circumstances the ability of a physician to defend against a malpractice claim may depend upon his ability to produce evidence establishing the patient's refusal of recommended treatment.

The patient's consent to an experimental procedure is an insufficient defense where the physician has deviated from the required standard of reasonable care and diligence or has undertaken a method of treatment which a reasonable practitioner would not have followed under the same circumstances. *Baldor* v. *Rogers*, 81 So.2d 658 (Fla. 1955); *Miller* v. *Toles*, 183 Mich. 252, 150N.W. 118 (1914); *Owens* v. *McCleary*, 313 Mo. App. 312, 281 S.W. 682 (1926); *McClarin* v. *Grenzfelder*, 147 Mo. App. 478, 126 S.W. 817 (1910); *Kershaw* v. *Tilbury*, 214, Cal. 679, iP.2d 109 (1932); *Graham* v. *Dr. Pratt Institute*, 163 Ill. App. 91 (1911).

Generally, drugs under clinical investigation should be administered only where: (1) the informed consent of the patient or his authorized representative has been obtained; (2) the physician is convinced of the reasonable accuracy of his diagnosis and, if necessary, has confirmed it by adequate consultation; and (3) existing methods of treatment have proven unsatisfactory. The voluntary participation of the patient will not excuse a deviation from the physician's obligation to exercise his best skill in rendering the care required of a reasonable practitioner. Furthermore, the physician is advised to confine his clinical investigations of new drugs to those furnished by reputable sources who have supplied him with comprehensive written information concerning: (1) animal experimentation; (2) previous clinical investigations, if any; (3) recommended dosages; (4) contraindications; (5) possible side-effects to be watched for; and (6) the safety and possible usefulness of thc drug, from existing data.

APPROACHES TO ACUPUNCTURE RESEARCH

Recommended By

The NIH Ad Hoc Committee on Acupuncture
July 17-18, 1972

It is likely that the most valuable first approach to a study of acupuncture would be in two areas:

I. SURGICAL ANESTHESIA

II. CERTAIN CHRONIC PAIN STATES

I. *SURGICAL ANESTHESIA*

The following data are needed in order to assess the feasibility of acupuncture anesthesia, and to understand something of its mechanism. It is presumed that these procedures will be carried out in the United States by investigators who have demonstrated by their training (a) that they have the ability to carry out research on this subject, (b) that they will investigate acupuncture anesthesia in the presence of full back-up equipment for chemical anesthesia in the event of failure of acupuncture, (c) that they will follow full ethical safeguards for the protection of experimental subjects.

The areas of research which should be encouraged are:

A. Complete clinical examination of patient under anesthesia.

—Neurological
—Autonomic, including respiration, hemodynamics, and G.I. state
—Metabolic and endocrine state
—Muscle relaxation
—Psychological state, including pain rating by point on agreed scale

B. Investigation of the factors influencing the patient's response.

—Relation to hypnotizability
—Role of training or preconditioning

—Role of relation between patient and physician
—Role of physician and the nature of his training
—Role of confusion, understanding, and age
—The effect of combined drug therapy and acupuncture

C. A study of the history of non-chemical methods of anesthesia.

D. A study of the social and economic factors of acupuncture anesthesia.

E. Further investigations on man under acupuncture anesthesia.

—Neurological, such as EEG, evoked potentials, depth recordings
—State of homeostatic mechanisms

F. A study of the state of animals under acupuncture anesthesia. This would require information from the Chinese about successful models which they have developed. It would require careful differentiation between animal hypnosis and specific acupuncture effects. The data needed would include:

—Neurological investigation, including depth recording
—Behavioral studies

G. Adequate clinical testing to define the essential factors.

—The importance of the exact point of needle insertion, and localization and size of effective area
—The influence of the patient's knowledge and beliefs
—The influence of the doctor's knowledge and beliefs
—The role of distant versus close needle insertion with relation to the points of incision
—The role of electrical stimulation close or far from the incision points
—Independent assessment of results

II. *CERTAIN CHRONIC PAIN STATES*

Here it would be necessary to study those states which present a well-defined clinical picture and have a predictable probability of continuance or remission. Examples would be neuralgias, reflex dystrophies, chronic visceral pain, cancer, and psychogenic pain.

A. The development of a therapeutic trial procedure in which:

—The patient is trained to describe his pain on a scale
—The effect of acupuncture is compared with other therapies
—Therapy is administered with suggestion or counter-suggestion
—Questioning of patient is conducted by independent observer
—The time course of the effect is recorded
—Studies are made of pre- and post-treatment activity and performance levels, e.g. specific exercise tolerances, and samples of daily activity schedules in relation to the reported pain states

B. Studies of the general state of patient under acupuncture therapy.

—Neurological
—Metabolic
—Psychological

C. Socio-economic studies of effectiveness of acupuncture analgesia.

D. Studies of personality and social environment of those patients who respond to therapy and those who do not, or who respond initially but who fail to react at later stages.

APPENDIX iii

EXCERPTS FROM ACUPUNCTURE UPDATE '74

(The following is the author's summary of "Acupuncture in Emergency Medicine" by Gerald Looney, M.D.)

Dr. Looney is professor of emergency medicine at the University of Southern California Medical School, and is affiliated with the Los Angeles County U.S.C. Medical Center. One of the largest medical centers in the world, its emergency department sees approximately 300,000 patients a year, or nearly 1,000 a day.

The average American, Dr. Looney points out, goes to an emergency room when in pain. More than 50 percent of emergency-room patients receive a prescription for some kind of analgesic. The center's decision to study acupuncture reflects this fact, as well as information that acupuncture is not only effective in reducing pain, but also of real benefit in acute emergency situations. Acupuncture in China is used by the "barefoot doctors" for on-the-scene emergency treatment, and an analogy exists between them and the U.S.C. paramedical staff. Finally, reports that acute musculo-skeletal pain—even fractures—may respond to acupuncture even better than chronic pain, needed practical substantiation.

In two years of studies some significant results emerged. When acupuncture points used by the Chinese to treat hemorrhagic shock were stimulated, blood flow in the opposite extremity dropped at least 24 percent, and in some patients as much as 56 percent. No change in blood flow occurred when acupuncture was used in pain or nonacupuncture sites.

Dr. Looney proposed a simple theory to explain the effects of acupuncture, much needed to overcome various professionals' opposition to this technique. His theory is based on a reevaluation of the role of the autonomic nervous system.

When acupuncture points are stimulated, either manually or electrically, a whole stream of autonomic stimuli (or at least afferent input) is introduced into the nervous system, which in turn causes a somato-sympathetic reflex. The remarkable specificity of this response is just being comprehended. Some laboratory examples of these effects, on both animals (who are of course not "suggestable") and humans, include:

- powerful reflex effects in the renal sympathetic when stimulating group-two afferents in the skin (Iwa and Mueller).
- reflex discharges in the splanchnic nerve trunk after stimulation of the superficial radial nerve (Miamoto and Allonis).
- electrical stimulation of visceral afferent fibers induced reflex discharges in the hypogastric nerve, and in sympathetic nerve branches going into the colon; but no reflex in the post-ganglionic fibers or the superior cervical ganglia.
- mass reflex discharges in the splanchnic nerves after tapping a cat's forelimb, or with vibrational stimuli to distal points of a man's arm.
- in man, painful electric stimuli to the ulna nerve triggered burst responses in presumably afferent fibers of the tibial nerve.
- distension of the pulmonary atrial junction increased discharge rates in the sympathetic fibers in cardiac nerves, decreased discharge rates in the renal sympathetic afference, and showed no effect on activity of the abdominal sympathetic trunk.

The therapeutic and motor effects observed with acupuncture are purely autonomic reflexes. Orthodox medical education, however, states that the autonomic nervous system is purely motor, with no relation to sensory functions. Dr. Looney's conviction is that this view of the autonomic nervous system is barely the tip of the iceberg. He suggests that the autonomic nervous system is very much involved with pain function and sensation; this is also suggested by the effects of sympathectomies on pain, and the Reilly Bay Syndrome, an autonomic malfunction characterized by the absence of pain perception. Acupuncture is thus seen as a key to unlocking secrets of the autonomic nervous system, in particular its relation to pain, pain perception, and pain generation.

ACUPUNCTURE IN OBSTETRICS

(The following information is from a lecture and series of audio-visual aids prepared by Charles Ledergerber, M.D., Clinical Assistant Professor at the University of California, Los Angeles School of Medicine.)

You may ask why I, as an obstetrician, ever got interested in acupuncture. My primary interest was pain relief—pain relief without doing any harm to mother and baby; pain relief without drugs with their side effects and allergies.

As an obstetrician, I've tried all my life to soften the fateful phrase from the Bible: "and, you shall bear children in labor and pain." The following are some perceptions I find useful:

POSSIBLE EXPLANATION OF ACUPUNCTURE

ELECTRICAL CHARGE UP	ELECTRICAL DISCHARGE
Stimulants, antidepressants Successful treatment by acupuncture of alcoholics & drug addicts (Dr. Wen Hsiang-Lai)	Alcohol, barbiturates, tranquilizers, marijuana, narcotics (Kirlian photography, Dr. Thelma Moss)
Successful treatment by acupuncture (Dr. Ledergerber, Dr. Gindes)	Impotence & frigidity (alcohol)
Routine acupuncture Electric generator (men—women)	A bath, overactivity, overeating, alcohol, drugs, fright and stress after acupuncture decrease the effects
Healer & acupuncturist transfer electric energy to patient	Treatment of disease & restoration of electric equilibrium
Heat, dryness (sunburn, heatstroke)	Cold, humidity (arthritis, rheumatism, cold, pneumonia, cystitis)
Chinese concept of semi-annual tune-up by acupuncture	Preventive medicine
Energy concept of life, soul, light, the universe and God	Disease, death, darkness

LABOR AND DELIVERY

1st Stage of Labor:

S_{44} or S_{36} ← electric current → Sp_6 uterine pain relief
Lv_2 Lv_3 ← electric current → B_{60} or B_{66} or B_{67} relieves pressure & backache
K_4 LI_4 B_2 LI_{20} GV_{26} Lv_8 P_7 optional

End of 1st, 2nd & 3rd Stages of Labor:

B_{21} B_{22} B_{23} relieves labor pains & backache (post. positions) lower dorsal & upper lumbar nerves (Bonica, Limoge)
B_{31} B_{32} B_{33} B_{34} for uterine & perineal anesthesia presacral & sacral nerves
CV_1 nature's own perineal acupuncture anesthesia
CV_2 CV_3 vaginal & perineal anesthesia
S_{29} or S_{30} needles directed into CV_2 } electric current
GV_2 GV_1 for rectal anesthesia } electric current

CAUTION: Too much current into B, Sp and CV meridian too close to the uterus produces stronger contractions

ELECTROACUPUNCTURE INDUCTION OF LABOR

Conception Vessel Meridian:

CV_5 strongest stimulator, forbidden point; CV_2 CV_3 CV_4 powerful stimulators

Spleen Meridian:

Sp_{15} very powerful stimulator; Sp_6 good stimulator

Bladder Meridian:

B_{66} B_{67} B_{60} good stimulators; B_{31} B_{32} B_{33} B_{34} powerful stimulators

Induction with current only: 200 mA at 12 Volts for 15 sec at 3-4 min interval

Induction with current & needles: 9-12 Volts 100-300 pulses per second

Pitocin & Tocosamine should not be used with needles & current in stimulating meridians close to the uterus → tetanic labor

Electric current potentiates & is potentiated by oxytocin. (Theobald) Electric current & pitocin may be used with electrostimulation without needles. Oxytocin may be used after electroacupuncture failure.

OLIGOMENORRHEA

Dr. Jean Claude Darras, Paris

I Physiological origin
II Psychological origin
III Hormonal origin

I OLIGOMENORRHEA PHYSIOLOGICAL ORIGIN

1. Anemia due to blood loss: Sp_2 Sp_3 Sp_{10} Lv_8 (B_{38} increases RBCs)
2. Nutritional anemia: Sp_3 Sp_6 S_{40} S_{36} CV_{12} Lv_3
3. Fatigue & exhaustion: Sp_8 B_{20} B_{49}
4. Renal insufficiency: CV_7 Sp_{10} B_{26}
5. Pelvic congestion: CV meridian Sp_2 Sp_4 Sp_6 Lv_2 K_2 S_{30}

II OLIGOMENORRHEA PSYCHOLOGICAL ORIGIN

1. Anxiety, headaches, estrasystolies: H_5 H_6 H_7 B_{44}
2. Dyspnea, facial congestion, asthma: SI_2 SI_3 H_7 H_9 L_8 L_{10}
3. Excessive sexual activity (vertigo, tinnitus, low backache): GB_{25} CV_1 CV_3 Sp_6 K_4 K_{10} B_{67}

III OLIGOMENORRHEA HORMONAL ORIGIN

1. Day 4-7: FSH & estrogen insufficiency: S_{28} S_{29} S_{30} LI_4 LI_{11} T_3
2. Day 14-21: LH insufficiency; B_{31} induces ovulation: GB_{28} GB_{41} T_5
3. Day 21-28: Progesteron insufficiency; premenstrual tension, migraines, breast engorgement: B_{23} B_{31} B_{32} B_{33} B_{34} GV_4 SI_3

AMENORRHEA OR OLIGOSPERMIA

All Points are Used Bilaterally

Dr. Bischko, Vienna; Dr. Ledergerber, Los Angeles

GB_3 Middle zygomatic bone

GV_{16} Base of skull action on pituitary gland

B_{31} Increases sperm count (Dr. Bischko)
Induces ovulation (Dr. Ledergerber) daily electroacupuncture from day 5-9 of menstrual cycle
Master point for menopause and dysmenorrhea

DYSMENORRHEA + PROSTATECTOMY PAIN

1. Dr. Bischko, Vienna
   B_{31} 1st sacral nerve
   GB_{26} GB_{28} Ilio-inguinal nerve
   GB_{34} Below knee, head of fibula controls muscular system
   CV_3 CV_4 CV_6
   Sp_6 Tender in dysmenorrhea and labor
   K_{11} Ilio-inguinal nerve
2. Dr. George Ulett
   Sp_4 Sp_6 Sp_{10} S_{36} S_{30} CV_4 LI_4 B_{20} Lv_5

HYPEREMESIS GRAVIDARUM

Dr. Bischko, Vienna

K_{21}
S_{21}
B_{39} Lateral scapula, 6th intercostal space

FRIGIDITY

Current ½ hour 5-6 weekly treatments

Points Used:

CV_3 CV_4 CV_6
Sp_6 Sp_{15}
B_{22} B_{23} B_{32} B_{60} → K_4 (Needle through Achilles tendon)
S_{36}

URINARY RETENTION

Dr. Guido Fisch
Lausanne, Switzerland

CV_2 CV_3
LI_1 LI_3 LI_8
S_{29} B_{64}
B_{23} B_{28} dilate urethra

(The following prescriptions are selected from the presentations of Drs. Ulett and Waylonis.)

HEADACHE — OCCIPITAL

Ulett
Bladder 10, 65
Small intestine 3
Large intestine 4
Gall bladder 20

Tan
Gall bladder 12, 20
Large intestine 4

HEADACHE — TEMPORAL

Ulett
Triple warmer 23
Gall bladder 4
Heart 8

Tan
Triple warmer 16, 22, 23
Ti-T'sang (corner mouth)
Large intestine 4

HEADACHE — FRONTAL

Ulett
- Large intestine 4
- Gall bladder 20
- Bladder 60

Tan
- Triple warmer 22
- Small intestine 18
- Large intestine 4, 18

HEADACHE — MIGRAINE

Willner
- Triple warmer 5
- Gall bladder 26
- Small intestine 1
- Gabella
- Heart 5
- Pericardium 7

Galliher
- Large intestine 4
- Circulation 7
- Spleen 36
- Liver 4, 8
- Kidney 10
- Lung 8
- Bladder 6, 7, 10
- Gall bladder 20
- Conception vessel 18

CERVICAL PAIN

Adel El-Etr
- Gall bladder 20
- Small intestine 11, 15
- Circulation 3
- Large intestine 4
- Triple warmer 15
- Conception vessel 13, 14, 16
- Bladder 11

Gencheff
- Small intestine 9, 15
- Gall bladder 20, 21
- Bladder 10, 11

Willner
- Large intestine 4
- Bladder 10
- Gall bladder 20

S. C. Mann
- Conception vessel 16
- Bladder 20
- Lung 2
- Gall bladder 21

THORACIC BACK PAIN

S.C. Mann
Conceptional vessel 9, 13
Bladder 11

Gencheff
Triggers
Gall bladder 20, 21

Tan
Trigger areas
Heart 8
Bladder 51

LOWER BACK PAIN

S.C. Mann
Conception vessel 2
Bladder 25, 28, 49, 54

Gencheff
Bladder 23, 30, 48, 49
Gall bladder 30
Sciatica: add Bladder 50, 51, 54, 57, 60

Tan
Bladder 35, 48, 49, 51, 53, 57
Gall bladder 36

SHOULDER PAIN

Adel El-Etr
Bladder 11, 12, 13
Triple warmer 3, 14
Small intestine 9
Large intestine 10

Tan
Large intestine 14, 15, 16
Small intestine 9, 10, 13
Lung 2
Gall bladder 34

S.C. Mann
Large intestine 15
Lung 2
Gall bladder 21
Triple warmer 14

Gencheff
Large intestine 4, 11, 14, 15, 16

ELBOW PAIN

S.C. Mann
- Large intestine 11
- Lung 5
- Heart 3
- Small intestine 8

Tan
- Large intestine 11, 12
- Small intestine 8
- Triple warmer 5

Gencheff
- Large intestine 4, 10, 11, 12

WRIST

S.C. Mann
- Large intestine 5
- Small intestine 5
- Triple warmer 4

Tan
- Triple warmer 4, 5
- Large intestine 5,6
- Lung 9

HAND—MP JOINT PAIN

S.C. Mann
- Large intestine 3
- Triple warmer 3
- Pericardium 8
- Heart 8

HIP

S.C. Mann
- Bladder 49
- Gall bladder 30

Tan
- Bladder 48, 49
- Gall bladder 30

Gencheff
- Gall bladder 30
- Bladder 50 (also 28, 29, 31)

KNEE

Willner
Gall bladder 34
Stomach 36
Liver 8

S.C. Mann
Spleen 9
Bladder 34
Stomach 34, 35, 43
Bladder 53

Galliher
Large intestine 4
Spleen 36
Heart 7, 8
Bladder 26
Kidney 2
Small intestine 2
Triggers

Tan
Stomach 34, 36
Gall bladder 34
Bladder 54

Gencheff
Stomach 34, 35, 36
\+ Triggers

FOOT PAIN (HEEL, SOLE)

Tan
Triggers
Spleen 6
Bladder 57

ANKLE PAIN

S.C. Mann
Gall bladder 40
Liver 4
Stomach 41
Kidney 5
Bladder 60

Tan
Stomach 41
Gall bladder 36, 40

COSTOCHRONDITIS

S.C. Mann
Lung 2
Stomach 17
Large intestine 12

INTERCOSTAL NEURALGIA

Galliher
- Circulation 5, 7
- Gall bladder 38
- Small intestine 5
- Lung 7
- Large intestine 4
- Spleen 36

TIC DOLOREUX

Galliher
- Small intestine 12, 13, 15, 16, 17, 18, 36*, 45*
- Bladder 1, 10
- Gall bladder 20

*Contralateral

Tan
- Bladder 2
- Small intestine 18, 19
- Stomach 4, 5, 44
- Large intestine 4
- Liver 2, 7

DEAFNESS

Morse
- Triple warmer 17, 21
- Small intestine 19
- Gall bladder 2

Tan
- Triple warmer 21
- Small intestine 19
- Gall bladder 2
- Conception vessel 19
- Large intestine 4, 18, 20
- Bladder 2

Galliher
- Conception vessel 2, 5, 10
- Lung 7
- Large intestine 4, 11
- Triple warmer 2, 3, 5, 16, 17, 18, 19, 20, 21
- Gall bladder 2, 25
- Small intestine 19
- Kidney 7
- Stomach 36
- Bladder 27, 67

HEMIPLEGIA (TAN)

Upper Extremity:
- Large intestine 4, 11, 15
- Triple warmer 5

Lower Extremity:
- Bladder 48, 59
- Gall bladder 31, 33, 36
- Liver 2

(ALL POINTS BILATERAL)

SOME HELPFUL ACUPUNCTURE FORMULAE

Seasonal Rhinitis			LI 21
or			LU 7
Chronic Vasomotor Rhinitis			LI 4
or			G 23
Acute Nasal Congestion			GB 20
			B 23
Tension Headaches	LI 4	SI 11	SI 15
	GB 20	SI 12	GB 21
	B 10	SI 14	LV 3
Dysmenorrhea		LU 7	K 15
		SPL 6	B 31
		LI 4	B 32
		STO 28	B 33
		LV 14	B 34
			G 12
Irregular Menses		SPL 6	C 6
		SPL 10	SPL 4
		STO 25	CX 6
		C 4	B 23
Prostatitis		G 1	B 32
		B 35	B 33
		B 31	B 34
Common Cold		B 12	B 13
		LI 4	
	(Add LU 11 for sore throat or tonsillitis)		
OR		LI 20	G 23
Tension Syndrome		G 4	STO 36
		G 20	SPL 6
		LI 4	LV 3
		H 7	G 26
Migraine Headaches		GB 20	GB 39
		B 10	LI 4
		G 16	S 36
		LV 3	LV 8

Tic (Facial Spasm)		Sedate	LI 4
		Sedate	STO 44
Male Impotence		B 31	B 23
		B 32	G 4
		B 33	
		B 34	
		B 47	
Tic Doloreux		GB 1	TH 17
		GB 2	SI 5
		GB 14	SI 6
		B 2	
Low Back Pain		Sedate	B 54
		plus local points	
Vomiting and Diarrhea		LI 4	
		STO 36	
		C 12	
Tennis Elbow		TH 10	
		LI 12	
		LI 10	
Nausea, Seasickness		B 10	
		TH 17	
Menorrhagia	SPL 1	LV 3	H 5
	C 6	B 55	STO 18
	H 1	B 54	SPL 2
Retained Placenta	GB 21	SPL 6	K 3
	B 67	B 47	B 32
	C 3	C 5	C 6
	C 7		

Warts—Needle in wart and then one on four sides of wart

Eclampsia	K 2	CX 7
	GB 21	GB 34
	SI 14	STO 36

To Induce Labor	Stimulate	LI 4
	Sedate	SPL 6

During Labor—B 28 at 45-degree angle into sacral foramen (2nd) directed caudally and distally. Use at point in labor when back pain is complained of. Keep in 15 minutes, twirled.

—C 4, C 2 (2″ needles) subcutaneously along linea alba, fully inserted directed caudally. This numbs perineum.

—PX 1, 3″ lateral to C 2, directed subcutaneously at 45-degree angle from vertical, toward vagina. This dilates cervix.

—Then use LI 4, SPL 6, STO 36 bilaterally.

Appetite Suppression	Sedate	STO 36
Cystitis	Sedate	B 62
	Sedate	K 8, 9, 10
Hot Flashes	Sedate	CX 6
	Sedate	SPL 10
Depression	Sedate	STO 36
	Stimulate	LI 11

INDEX